THE PUBLIC'S
HEALTH

A NARRATIVE HISTORY OF
HEALTH AND DISEASE IN ARKANSAS

BY SAM TAGGART, M.D.

PUBLISHED BY ARKANSAS TIMES

TABLE OF
CONTENTS

ACKNOWLEDGEMENTS

If it had not been for Amanda Saar, the librarian at the Historical Research Center of the University of Arkansas Medical Center Library, this book would not have gotten done. Also greatly appreciate the assistance of April Brooks and Suzanne Easley of the HRC; Steve Perdue, the county historian at the Saline County Library in Benton; the staff at the Butler Center for Arkansas Studies; the staff of the Arkansas Department of Health: Ed Barham, Dr. Dirk Haselow, Dr. Bill Mason, Dr. Glen Baker, Paul Halverson Ph.D., John Senner, Dr. Joseph H. Bates, Mary Gaither, PHN; and Dr. Tom Bruce and Dr. Steve Collier for their insights on rural health. A special thanks to Will Taggart for research at Emory University. Thanks to Bill Simmons of Benton and Marilyn Cox of Benton.

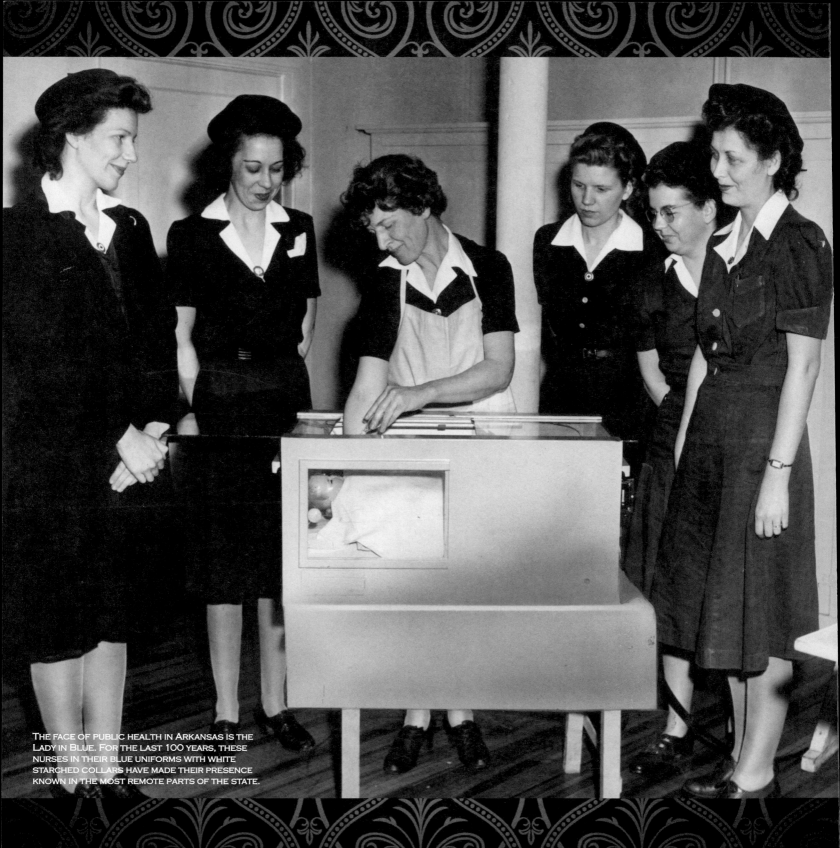

THE FACE OF PUBLIC HEALTH IN ARKANSAS IS THE LADY IN BLUE. FOR THE LAST 100 YEARS, THESE NURSES IN THEIR BLUE UNIFORMS WITH WHITE STARCHED COLLARS HAVE MADE THEIR PRESENCE KNOWN IN THE MOST REMOTE PARTS OF THE STATE.

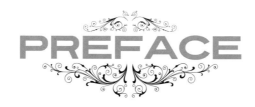

PREFACE

BY JOSEPH H. BATES, M.D.

The year 2013 marks the 100th anniversary of the Arkansas Department of Health. Its creation by the Arkansas Legislature in 1913 was a result of protracted efforts by Governors Donaghey and Robinson, together with many community leaders and organizations, in particular, the Women's City Club. It will come as no surprise to those interested in Arkansas politics and history that many well-known leaders in the state legislature and community were opposed to establishing a new agency of state government with some degree of control over their lives. Arkansans of the day were suspicious of most governmental organizations and preferred as little government regulation as possible.

Once created, the Health Department faced a daunting set of health challenges. No official records were kept regarding details of births and deaths. There were very few hospitals and most illnesses, no matter how serious, were cared for in the home. Almost all surgery was done in the home on the kitchen table with little regard for sterile technique. Pregnancy was a serious health threat, and one pregnant woman in 100 died either during pregnancy or soon after delivery. The chance of a newborn infant dying in the first year of life was 1 in 5, and if he survived the trials of the first year he could only expect to live to be 47 years old.

In the early 1900s, the most common illnesses and causes of death were tuberculosis, pneumonia, malaria, typhoid fever and dysentery. One child in 5 had hookworm infection, a serious debilitating infection. These constant life-threatening illnesses, for which there was little or no treatment, were punctuated by epidemics of cholera and yellow fever that would cause a surge in deaths, creating great difficulties for struggling small towns and cities.

In 1900, unsafe drinking water was the source of dysentery, cholera and typhoid fever. Waste water, dead animals and sewage were dumped into small streams or rivers, including the Arkansas River, and then these same rivers were used as a source of water for human consumption and bathing. Indoor plumbing and sanitary sewer systems were unknown. Today, more than 90 percent of all Arkansans enjoy properly chlorinated, high quality drinking water provided by 1,100 public water systems, all regulated by Health Department staff.

In the early years of the Health Department, there was an effort to reduce the threat of smallpox that took the lives of so many each year. By 1920, the smallpox vaccine was available and Arkansas was one of the first states to require that all children be vaccinated against smallpox before enrolling in school. Predictably, there was stiff opposition to such a mandate: it was contested in the courts until finally the Arkansas Supreme Court upheld the rule. As a result the number of smallpox cases fell to zero. Gradually, the state immunization program expanded to bring under control and almost eliminate other serious diseases, including measles, whooping cough, mumps, and polio. Even today, sadly, the use of vaccines to prevent these dreaded diseases is opposed by a few outspoken persons who challenge the safety of vaccines.

Without question, the provision of safe drinking water is a major achievement of public health in the first 100 years, closely followed by proper management of waste water, major advances in maternal and child health and the development of a state wide network of well-regulated hospitals that provide quality care for all. Taken together, these advances, along with many others in clinical medicine, have added 33 years to the life expectancy of Arkansans and 25 of these years are a result of public health achievements.

As readers turn the pages of this narrative they will be amazed and entertained to learn of the battles, victories, dramas, and steady progress that evolved to improve and protect the health of all Arkansans.

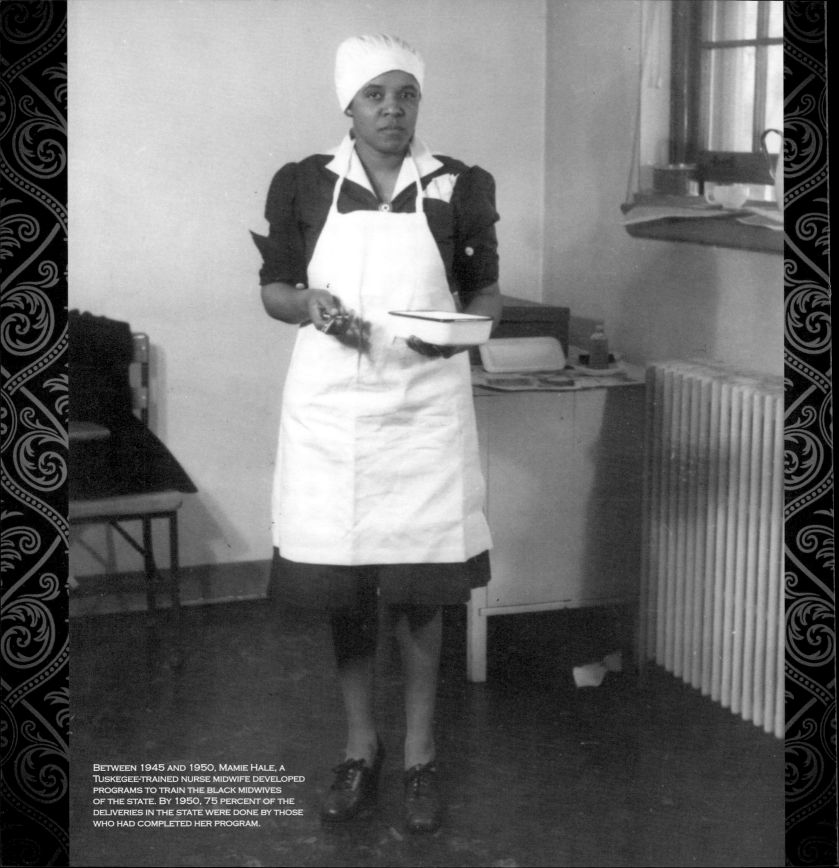

Between 1945 and 1950, Mamie Hale, a Tuskegee-trained nurse midwife developed programs to train the black midwives of the state. By 1950, 75 percent of the deliveries in the state were done by those who had completed her program.

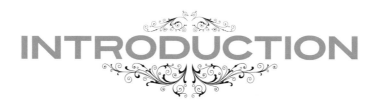

INTRODUCTION

"As the woman in white, with her technical terms,
soothes the brow and counts out the pills;
her sister in blue wages her fight with germs
in the swamps and the hills."

Excerpt from The Women in Blue by Maggie White, Public Health Nurse, Bradley County Health Unit, 1945

The face of public health in Arkansas is the Lady in Blue. For the last 100 years these nurses in their blue uniforms and white starched collars have made their presence known in the most remote parts of the state. There is a cadre of these women whose names appear and reappear throughout the century; Linnie Beauchamp is an excellent example. The daughter of a physician from Wheatley, Arkansas, she was the first official public health nurse of the State Board of Health in 1918. In 1950, when the State Polio Committee was formed, she and Mary Emma Smith, also a retired public health nurse, took on the task of training nurses how to deal with these sick and paralyzed children. When Adolphine Terry created the Women's Emergency Committee to Open Our Schools in response to the desegregation crisis in 1958, Linnie Beauchamp's name was on the committee's list of signees.

Whether these women were dealing with tuberculosis, malaria, smallpox, polio, angry physicians or uncooperative legislators, it is their faces that bring forth the most persistent memories of public health: the nurse who came to the school to give polio shots; the hospice nurse who took care of grandma when she was dying; the TB nurse who helped get an old uncle into the Booneville Sanatorium; the lady who subbed as the sanitation expert, checking the outdoor privy and taking water samples; the nice lady who handed out WIC food supplies so a kid could eat; the nurse who admonished the children to get a typhoid shot before swimming in the river.

At the beginning of the 20th century tuberculosis ravaged the state of Arkansas. The earliest public health nurses were first sent into homes in Jackson County to search for those who were plagued with consumption. These nurses had almost no resources and were dependent on the kindness of county judges to help provide a place to work, funding and moral support. The Red Cross, the Arkansas Tuberculosis Association and the Arkansas Federation of Women's Clubs stood behind these ladies and often provided powerful lobbying support.

Each decade of the 20th century presented these storm troopers with new challenges. In the 1910s, they faced tuberculosis, hookworm, malaria, syphilis and a pandemic of Spanish flu. In the 1920s, they uncovered widespread malnutrition, high infant mortality rates and, in 1927, they were confronted with a catastrophic flood. The 1930s brought the Depression and drought with starvation; these were followed by another major flood in 1937. As life expectancy began to increase, the 1940s saw the emergence of heart disease, stroke and cancer as the principal sources of death and disability. In the 1950s, the plague of polio captured the attention of everyone in the state; it was the duty of public health nurses not just to deal with the acute paralytic disease of polio but the crippled children who were left in its wake. The 1960s, 1970s and 1980s saw major inroads into maternal, infant and childhood problems: family planning, prenatal care, nutrition, health education and mass immunization occupied a good deal of their time. Since 1990 AIDS, childhood obesity and the disparities of minority and rural health have been a major focus of the nurses who man the local health units across the state.

For most of the 20th century these nurses worked for the Arkansas Board of Health. In the late 19th century there were a series of temporary and unofficial boards but in 1913 the first permanent Arkansas State Board of Health was created. However, that isn't where our story begins. Our story begins in 1804 with the beginning of the public in Arkansas. At the turn of the 19th century there were less than 3,000 people living in what became the state of Arkansas. Despite its isolation, by 1913 the state's population had mushroomed to 1.6 million and to 3 million in 2013.

Before beginning the narrative of health and disease of Arkansas, we will touch briefly on the geography and climate and the effect they have on the health of the state. In addition, we will explore the demise of the American Indian population of the state which set the stage for the influx of white European settlers.

When writing a history of the public's health in Arkansas it would be easy to get lost in the facts and figures, the statistics of death and disease; but, the real story of the public's health is the story of the people of Arkansas, what they faced and how they responded.

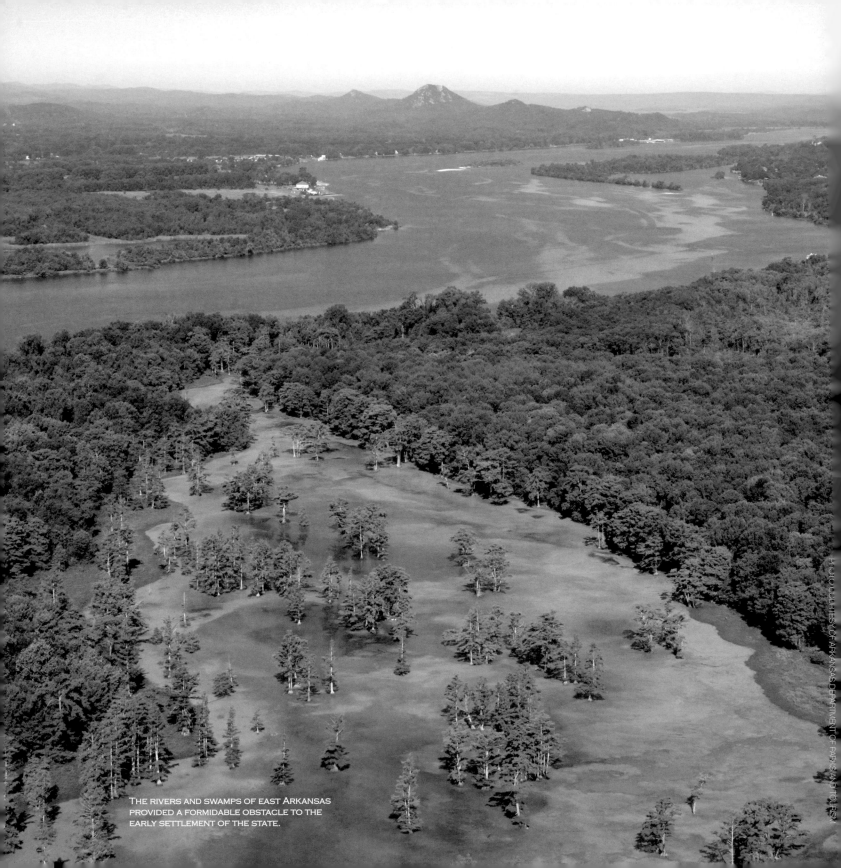

THE RIVERS AND SWAMPS OF EAST ARKANSAS
PROVIDED A FORMIDABLE OBSTACLE TO THE
EARLY SETTLEMENT OF THE STATE.

CHAPTER ONE
THE LAY OF THE LAND

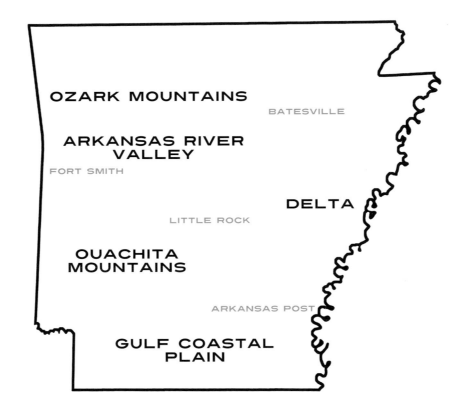

As in any good story the place becomes a key element, the stage on which the story evolves. In these pages the place we call Arkansas is one of the central characters. Not only is it where all the action takes place, the physical being of Arkansas changes as the story proceeds. At any one time we may see the face of rich river bottomland that invites farming, beautiful mountain tops that inspire the soul, hot springs that heal the sick or abundant fish and game that sustain people during times of need. If we turn away and then look back we will see prolonged droughts, the devastation of massive flooding, life changed in an instant by violent tornadoes or the land sinking and rivers running backward. In all of these scenes the mere humans follow its lead.

To tell the tale of health and disease in Arkansas, we must first talk a bit about climate and the lay of the land.

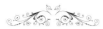

Harry Ashmore, former editor of the *Arkansas Gazette*, once described Arkansas as "the boundaries of a vast game preserve."

Harry Ashmore, former editor of the *Arkansas Gazette*, once described Arkansas as "the boundaries of a vast game preserve." The western part of the state is largely rugged mountains with free flowing, clear water streams. When the European settlers first arrived, bison, elk, deer, cougar and black bear roamed the mountains and hollows of the western part of the state. Most of the river delta lands in the eastern part of the state were dominated by dense hardwood forests, swamps and slow moving rivers. The state is in the middle of the Mississippi flyway for migratory birds; on a clear day in December the skies are black with ducks and geese. The slow moving streams and oxbow lakes of east Arkansas are always full of fish. The state is dotted with springs that provide clear good tasting water and many have been touted for their therapeutic value. The topsoil in the delta is exceptionally rich; the old joke in east Arkansas is that you can tickle the ground and it will cough up a crop. It is the moderate climate and the lay of the land that explains this abundance.

The state sits squarely in the middle of the North American Continent and all of the major rivers between the Appalachians on the east and the Rockies to the west converge at or near the state. The Mississippi River forms the eastern border and its delta lands make up a third of the state. Because of millennia of regular flooding, the topsoil in the eastern half of the state is said to be 50-plus feet deep in places making it some of the richest land in the world. For the early settlers the other side to this two-edged sword was the nearly impenetrable swamps and mosquitoes. These swamps created a barrier and limited the exploration, settlement and development of Arkansas for several centuries. Bob Lancaster, in his book, *The Jungles of Arkansas*, quotes an unknown early explorer who got lost in the swamps of the Delta, wandering out several weeks later, desperately fending off the mosquitoes saying, "Arkansas could not be a place for which Jesus Christ died." The Arkansas River courses west to east across the state dividing the Ozark Mountains in the north and west from the Ouachita Mountains in the south. Like the Mississippi, the Arkansas River has a broad fertile valley. It has many areas of rich deep topsoil and because of accumulated sediment and plant life in the valley and eons of time, the buried plant life has been converted into coal and natural gas. The south central part of the state is dominated by the Gulf Coastal Plain. In the distant past it was a series of shallow off-shore reefs and when the waters of the Gulf receded it left behind sand, clay, gravel and silt; these areas became grasslands and woodlands. Another interesting aspect of the Gulf Coastal Plain is the deposits of salt left behind when the sea receded. A number of the springs that percolate up through the ground are sources of salt that have been mined and used for human consumption.

The sub-tropical climate with 50 inches of rain a year, hot humid summers and mild to cool winters complement the variety of terrain and natural resources.

With that said, the stage is set for the humans to enter.

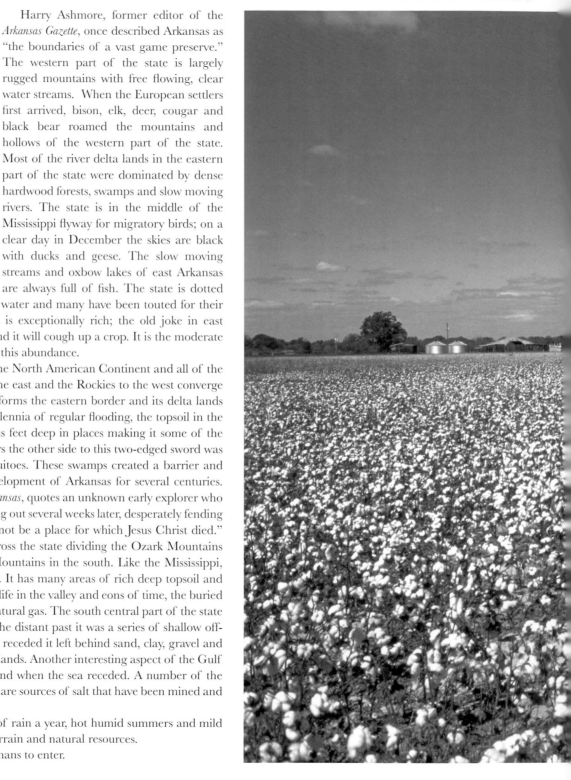

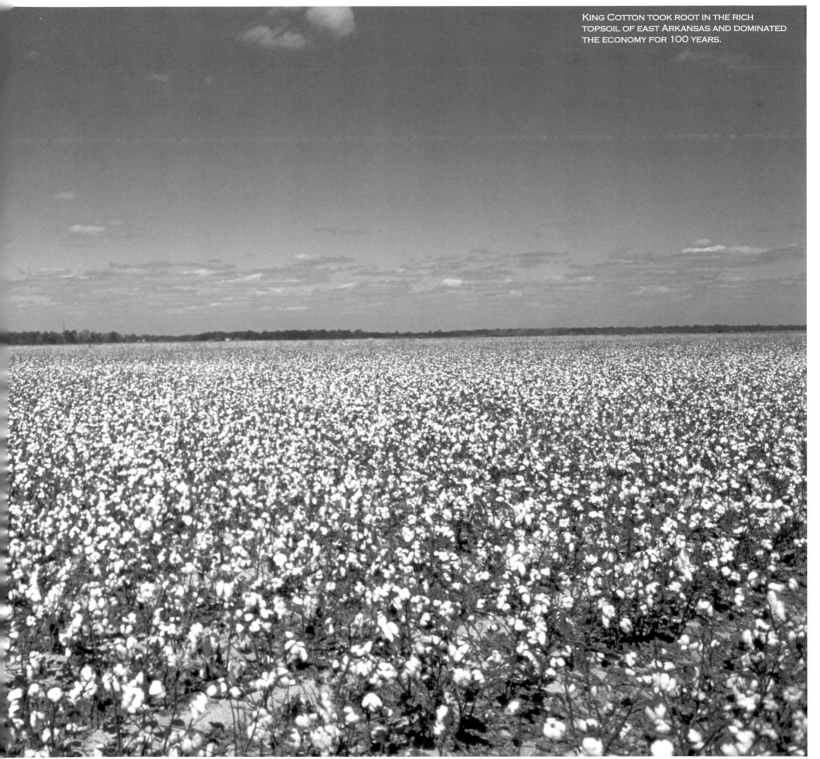

KING COTTON TOOK ROOT IN THE RICH
TOPSOIL OF EAST ARKANSAS AND DOMINATED
THE ECONOMY FOR 100 YEARS.

PHOTO COURTESY OF ARKANSAS DEPARTMENT OF PARKS AND TOURISM

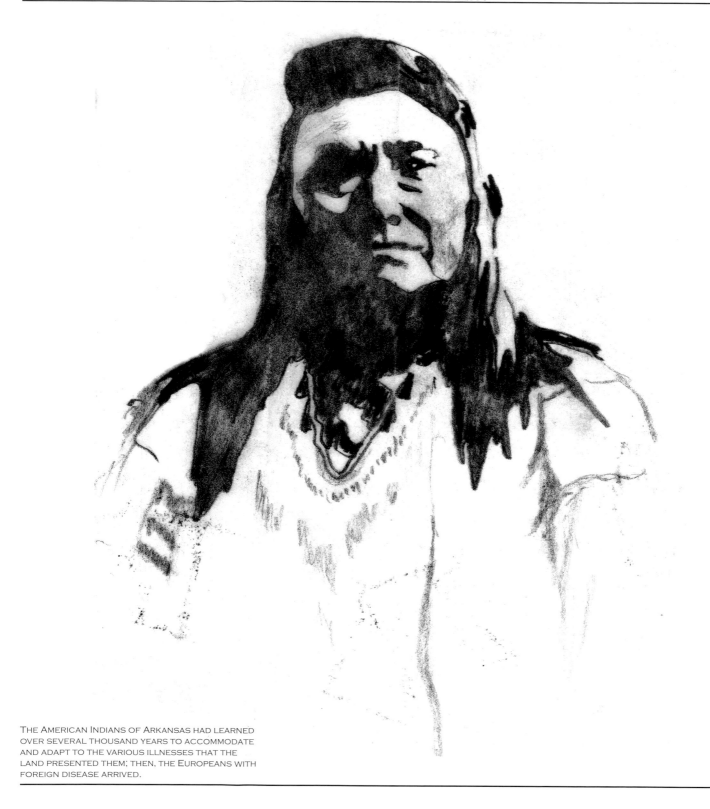

THE AMERICAN INDIANS OF ARKANSAS HAD LEARNED
OVER SEVERAL THOUSAND YEARS TO ACCOMMODATE
AND ADAPT TO THE VARIOUS ILLNESSES THAT THE
LAND PRESENTED THEM; THEN, THE EUROPEANS WITH
FOREIGN DISEASE ARRIVED.

CHAPTER TWO
OUR PREDECESSORS

Thirteen thousand years ago humans entered the Mississippi River Valley. There is good evidence that these early people followed the woolly mammoth and mastodons into the region, setting up seasonal hunting camps near the routes taken by the large animals. Over several millennia these camps became permanent. Their cultures slowly evolved and eventually they made the switch from hunter-gatherer to agricultural societies based primarily in the river valleys. Since there were no written languages among these peoples, we know little about them except that like most civilizations they rose and fell. There is good evidence that several of these cultures were quite sophisticated and had extensive trade across large areas of the North American continent. Poverty Point in northeast Louisiana was a vibrant trading center and around 2,600 years ago was simply abandoned.

At the time of first European contact in 1541, there were substantial populations of mound-building chiefdoms living across the territory. The largest number appeared to have lived in the delta of east Arkansas near the Mississippi, White and St. Francis rivers. The first 100 years after European contact represents a black hole in the history of Arkansas. When the next Europeans descended the Mississippi 100 years later, they discovered only a small number of American Indians, Quapaw and Mitchigamea. These tribes insisted they had moved down from the Ohio River valley and taken land from the Tunica Indians.

The question arises: Why did these people, many who had lived here for thousands of years, leave? This question has been a matter of speculation and disagreement for the last several centuries.

In 1984 at the Southeastern Archeological Society Meeting in Florida, Archeologist John House presented evidence that the St Francis River area was abandoned between the years 1550 to 1560 CE; this would have been 10 years after Desoto's visit. House speculates that their culture fell secondary to malnutrition. His reasoning is that their reliance on corn as a mainstay in their diet had resulted in problems with iron deficiency anemia. It does not seem reasonable that these peoples who had evolved in this environment for as many as 10,000 years, had been consuming corn for 1,200-1,500 years and

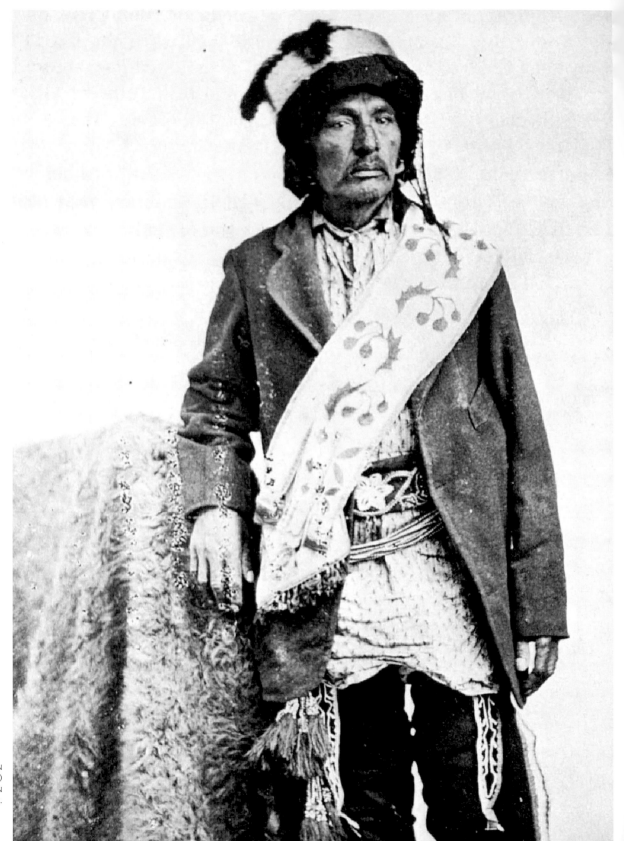

CADDO GEORGE WASHINGTON
(OR SHO-E-TAT, LITTLE BOY)
DRESSED AS BEFITS HIS POSITION
AS A CADDO CHIEF.

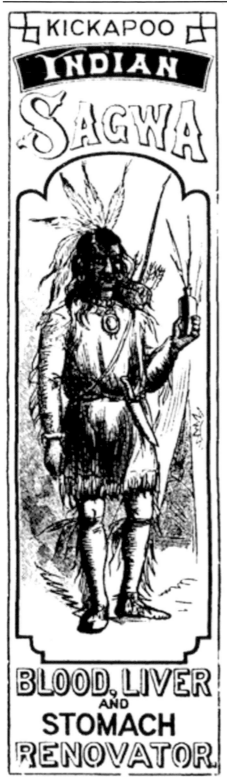

had complex dietary patterns would have failed in this fashion. Almost no one gives credence to this idea as the principal reason for their disappearance.

It is possible that severe floods and droughts could have forced them to move on. It is reported that when Desoto and his men made their trip through the country it was in the midst of a severe drought.

The American Indians who lived in the Mississippi Valley were not the idyllic peace lovers written about in early text books; like man everywhere they engaged in war. They tended to be tightly bound to family group and the leaders of their group. They fought over access to hunting areas, land for cultivation and in some cases just for dominance. With few exceptions this was not the type of warfare where everyone including women and children were stricken from the face of the earth.

Communities of American Indians had been known to move lock, stock and barrel after an epidemic of disease. There is a suggestion that the Quapaw moved from their home on the Ohio River because of an epidemic of smallpox in the late 16th century.

Even though we do not have direct written documentation about the territory of Arkansas we do know what was going on in the rest of the country and it seems reasonable to assume that Arkansas and its native populations were not spared. Starting in the 1520s and extending through the Colonial period and beyond, periodic epidemics plagued the indigenous people of the Western Hemisphere. Smallpox and measles were the first and most devastating. The epidemics occurred everywhere the European soldiers went.

The American Indians had learned over several thousand years to accommodate and adapt to the various illnesses that the land presented to them. When the Europeans arrived they brought with them a number of diseases that were endemic in Europe and Africa. The native populations had no immunity to these illnesses such as smallpox, measles, yellow fever, malaria, typhoid, cholera, and flu. Several of these illnesses, especially the mosquito-borne diseases of malaria and yellow fever became endemic in parts of the American south. With minimal contact, these devastating illnesses went through virgin communities like wildfire. Estimates are that 80 to 90 percent of the native populations in the United States were killed off in less than one hundred years by disease. Despite the fact that Arkansas was somewhat isolated from much of the rest of the North American continent there were extensive foot paths that led from one region to another and the rivers were navigable most of the year. It is reasonable to assume that they suffered the same fate as those in the rest of the country.

The written records that do exist after the mid-17th century show that there was an epidemic of some description among the American Indian populations every four to five years during the 17th and 18th centuries.

When the land that would be Arkansas was transferred to the United States in 1804 there were very few people—less than 500 white Europeans and their slaves and 1,500 to 2,000 American Indians. Because all of those who lived in the territory were in scattered small groups exact figures are difficult to determine; however, the territory of Arkansas was most certainly a frontier.

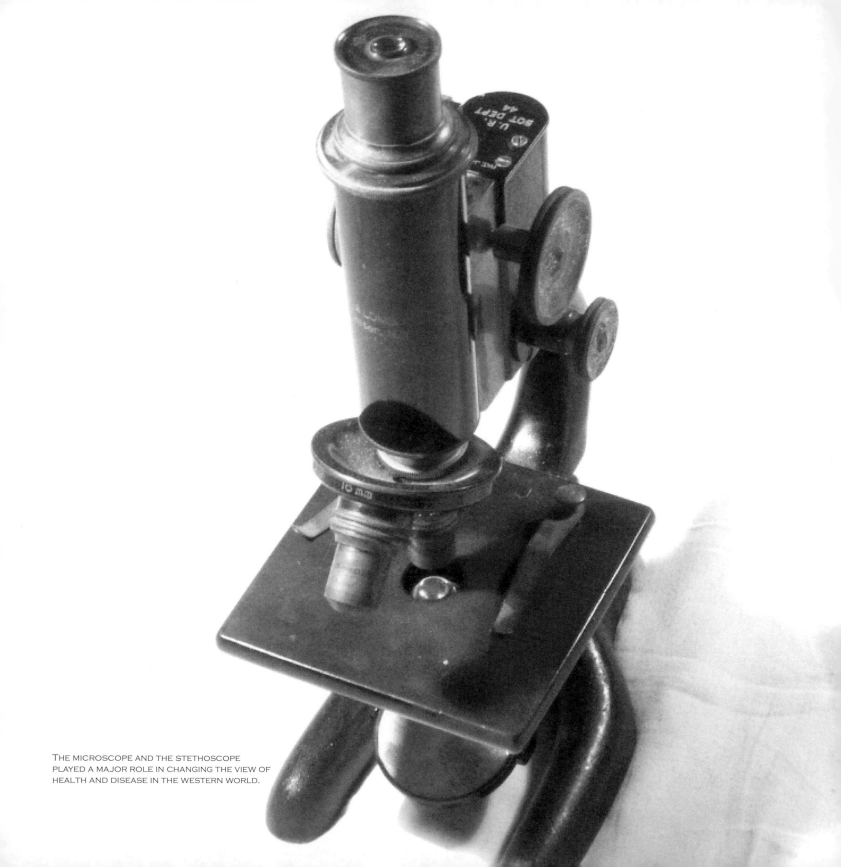

THE MICROSCOPE AND THE STETHOSCOPE
PLAYED A MAJOR ROLE IN CHANGING THE VIEW OF
HEALTH AND DISEASE IN THE WESTERN WORLD.

CHAPTER THREE
STARTING FROM SCRATCH

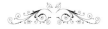

In 1804, William Hix opened a ferry across the Current River in what is now northeast Randolph County on the Southwest Trail and put up a sign that read: "Welcome to the Gateway of Arkansas."

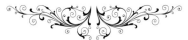

With the Louisiana Purchase in 1804 the United States took possession of the territory that would be Arkansas. In the early part of the century, Arkansas was to be part of the land that would be ceded to the Indians in exchange for their lands in the eastern United States. The government didn't really know what it had purchased from France, and it took several expeditions along the Mississippi, Missouri, Arkansas and Red Rivers before the extent of the Louisiana Purchase was known. For the first decade in-migration was slow for the same reasons that the French and Spanish had not flocked to Arkansas: the land was inhospitable; mosquitoes and disease such as intermittent fevers (malaria) were fierce.

Prior to the War of 1812, there was the constant possibility of conflict in addition to uncertain Spanish, French and Indian land claims. After the war, migration began in earnest. The initial routes of exploration were along the waterways because the land routes required braving the swamps of east Arkansas. The one exception was an old Indian trail that came to be known as the Southwest Trail or the Old Military Road. It followed a foot path 10 to 15 miles up in the hills from the northeast corner to the southwest corner of the state, avoiding the low lands to the east and at the same time mosquitoes. In 1804, William Hix opened a ferry across the Current River in what is now northeast Randolph County on the Southwest Trail and put up a sign that read: "Welcome to the Gateway to Arkansas." Other than Arkansas Post at the mouth of the Arkansas and White Rivers and a small community across the river from Memphis, Tennessee, called Hopefield, most of the early communities in Arkansas were along the Southwest Trail: Davidsonville on the Black River, Poke Bayou (Batesville) on the White River as it emerged from the mountains, Cadron on the Arkansas River (slightly north of modern Conway), Little Rock on the Arkansas River as it entered the delta lands, Saline Crossing (Benton) on the Saline River and Old Washington near the Red River in the southwest corner of the state. Most of these communities were nothing more

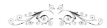

Archibald Yell, the second governor of Arkansas, said of the citizens of Arkansas, "...every man left his honesty and every woman left her chastity on the other side of the Mississippi."

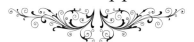

than way-stations—a post office, rooming house, saloon and supply house often in the same building. Ninety-five percent of the population lived in the country and were quite isolated. Fort Smith on the Arkansas River began as a military post on the Western border of the state and soon established itself as an economic center based on the military and trade with the Indians. Throughout the Colonial Period and the early territorial years Arkansas Post was the administrative center of the region. It was plagued by flooding, mosquitoes and disease; in 1820 the capital was moved to Little Rock in the center of the territory.

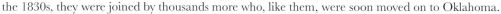

WHO WERE THE FIRST OF THESE NEW WAVES OF IMMIGRANTS AND WHAT DID THEY FACE?

The Quapaw had gradually lost most of their numbers to war and pestilence; they never regained any of their population, and after several moves, all of which were unsuccessful, they ceded their lands and were removed to Eastern Oklahoma. The Osage Indians from Missouri Territory made forays into northern Arkansas for the purposes of hunting but did not have a permanent presence. In the first third of the 19th century American Indian tribes from the eastern United States partially filled the void: the Cherokee, the Choctaw and the Chickasaw made their presence known in Arkansas for short periods of time. The largest of the groups who lived in Arkansas were the Cherokee who settled first in the St. Francis bottomland of east Arkansas in 1780 and then after the New Madrid Earthquake of 1812 moved to west central Arkansas north of Morrilton and Russellville. During the Indian removal of the 1830s, they were joined by thousands more who, like them, were soon moved on to Oklahoma.

As had been true under the French and the Spanish there were trappers, hunters and river men who came to the frontier to escape the pressures of an increasing dense population east of the Mississippi. In general they were a rough cut of people best described by our second governor, Archibald Yell, when he said, "every man left his honesty and every woman her chastity on the other side of the Mississippi."

Military and professional men were sent by Washington to help explore and administer the new territory. The first territorial governor, James Miller, came and went in a short period of time, and most of the time he was sick with "ague and fever." The first governor of the state, James Conway, came to Arkansas as a land surveyor and settled near what would be the town of Bradley in Lafayette County. At least one territorial judge in 1820 made his way to Arkansas Post, was attacked by a swarm of mosquitoes and left on the next boat out. In 1828 Superior Court Judge Thomas P. Elkridge came for one season and never returned. Instead he sent a note from his doctor explaining why he could not stay in the state. It read in part: "It is conceived impossible for you to return to Arkansas until, by an absence of another summer, you shall enjoy the advantage of another year, of restoring the healthy condition of your liver." The doctor's note was published in the *Arkansas Gazette.*

The majority of the first immigrants were poor young men looking for a piece of good land that was unclaimed. Often they came alone, cleared a plot of land, built a house and then sent for their family.

As to what these adventurous souls faced, it was clearly a hard life. Basic food staples like flour and salt were only intermittently available. In the 1820s mining of salt springs in the Ouachita Mountains and Arkansas River Valley became a reliable source of salt. Most of the basic needs that required importing came first by river and hand-powered keel boats; in the days before steamboats this was quite unpredictable. Even after the advent of steamboats, the rivers regularly flooded or drought dropped the water levels so low that the boats could not navigate; in either case the rivers were mine fields of sandbars and uprooted trees. Most of the exotic supplies like tea, coffee, sugar, bluing dye, soda and spices came up river from New Orleans. Flour and other supplies came down river from the Ohio River. Throughout the first half of the 19th century there are newspaper articles referring to the scarcity of flour and other basic food stuffs. The principal meat sources were pork and wild

Superior Court Judge Thomas P. Elkridge came for one season and never returned. Instead he sent a note from his doctor explaining why he could not stay in the state. It read in part: "It is conceived impossible for you to return to Arkansas until, by an absence of another summer, you shall enjoy the advantage of another year, of restoring the healthy condition of your liver."

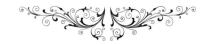

game. Taking a page from the Indians, homegrown corn, beans and squash were common staples in the settler's diet. Despite using corn as a mainstay in their diet the settlers did not adopt the Indian nixtamalization of corn. Over several thousand years the American Indians had learned that cooking corn with ash killed the seed, prevented it from sprouting in storage and made the corn a more complete food. In the 20th century nutritional chemists would determine that the nixtamalization process freed the Vitamin B-3 (niacin) that was bound in the grain making it more bioavailable. Without this process, a form of malnutrition called pellagra is a real possibility. Pellagra became a major disease problem in Arkansas and the rest of the South. It was never adequately dealt with until the Flood of 1927. By the middle decades of the 19th century, sorghum molasses had been added to this dietary mix. Bee hives were kept and honey was a staple of the diet. The basic diet was characterized as the 3-M diet: meat, meal and molasses.

CONTAGIONISTS VS. ANTI-CONTAGIONISTS AND MALARIA

As to the health problems they faced and how they dealt with them, it is important to remember that the medical professionals of the early 19th century were of two minds about disease—the contagionists and the anti-contagionists. For two millennia health and disease in Western culture had been dominated by Galen's Theory of Four Humors. According to this theory, the body was composed of four humors: black bile, yellow bile, phlegm and blood. Most disease especially those of internal origin were considered to be either a disturbance of one or more of these humors or a form of divine retribution as a result of sin. An illness was described by the principal symptom it created, and no attempt was made to differentiate between the root causes.

Most major disease and especially those of an epidemic nature were thought to be caused by a constellation of weather conditions and local circumstances. Hippocrates wrote about weather changes and the nature of seasons affecting the rise and fall of epidemics. This gave rise to the idea of an epidemic constitution of a location that must exist for an epidemic to develop, and as long as it was in place the disease or epidemic of disease would continue. The word malaria is derived from the Latin word for malodorous air, miasma. For centuries it had been noticed that low areas that flooded where decaying matter was allowed to accumulate created malodorous air, bred disease and intermittent fevers.

It was this theory of the miasmatic origin of most epidemic illness that dominated up through the mid-19th century. Even though the premise for the theory proved to be wrong, the sanitation movement of the 19th century derived some of its impetus to clean up cities in Europe and the United States from the idea of disease emanating from filth.

In opposition to the miasmatic theories were the contagionists who contended that there was a contagion that was responsible for the rise and spread of epidemic disease. As early as the mid-16th century, Girolamo Fracastoro presented a paper, "On Contagion, Contagious Diseases" and their treatment, where he outlined the theory of infection as we understand it today. He contended that epidemic disease was caused by minute infective agents that are transmissible and self-propagating. It is unlikely he thought of these agents as living organisms but more like chemical substances or ferments. After studying several different diseases including the plague and typhus, he concluded that illnesses were propagated through direct human-to-human contact, through intermediate agents or through the air. His theory completed with the miasmatic theory until the advent and proof of the germ theory in the last half of the nineteenth century.

In 1676, Antony van Leeuwenhoek, a linen draper and microscopist, presented a letter to the Royal Society in London describing a series of little animals that he had observed under his microscope; he described these organisms as cocci, rods and spirilla based on their shape. No attempt was made to relate these to disease but near this same time Athanasius Kircher, a Jesuit, made an explicit claim of observing a living organism as the cause of plague. His theories received some support, but because the technology was

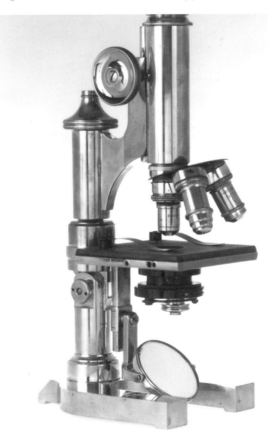

IN 1676, ANTONY VAN LEEUWENHOEK, A LINEN DRAPER AND MICROSCOPIST, PRESENTED A LETTER TO THE ROYAL SOCIETY IN LONDON DESCRIBING A SERIES OF "LITTLE ANIMALS" THAT HE HAD OBSERVED UNDER HIS MICROSCOPE. HE DESCRIBED THESE ORGANISMS AS COCCI, RODS AND SPIRILLA BASED ON THEIR SHAPE.

"It is evident that, at times, certain atmospheric conditions, contain exhalations from the soil and certain electrical states concur and form an epidemic constitution through which agency a morbid poison propagates itself with unusual rapidity and intensity. The disease may be common marsh fever, yellow fever, bubo-plague or cholera depending on the circumstance of locality and habitat."

Dr. A.W. Webb

poor, attempts to confirm his work were confusing and contradictory; this created a reaction against the germ theory of disease.

Even if the scientific community did not fully accept the contagious nature of most epidemic disease, large parts of the general public did, and they generally voted with their feet. Epidemics such as the plague, typhus, smallpox and measles sent people running to the hills. Well before the germ theory was formulated or proven the idea of isolation and quarantine were widely accepted practices. The ancient shunning of lepers was an example of the belief in the effectiveness of limiting the spread of an infectious disease.

To paint a picture of all or none is not accurate, by the beginning of the 19th century many of the university-trained physicians in Europe and the United States had a foot in both camps. In part because neither contagion nor anti-contagion theory fully accounted for all of the problems associated with epidemic disease. It was clear that healthcare workers could work among those with cholera and not get the disease—assuming they did not drink the same water. Those working with yellow fever did not necessarily get the fever unless they were bitten by the mosquitoes. On the other side of the coin, smallpox attacked regardless of the environmental conditions.

As early as 1873, well before the germ theory was accepted as fact, an Arkansas physician, Dr. D.H Dungan, writing for the "Report of the Board of Health on Cholera" in Little Rock and speaking of the housing on a plantation south of Little Rock said, "the houses with their surroundings present about as inviting a prospect to infectious germs that seek pabulum whereon to feed as can well be imagined."

The death knell for the miasmatic theory was sounded in 1840 by Jacob Henle, a young professor of Anatomy at Zurich. In a paper published in Berlin, he formulated a theory that living microscopic organisms were the cause of contagious and infectious disease. This and other reports he published set the stage for the work of Pasteur, Lister and Koch in the second half of the 19th century and the rise of bacteriology and immunology.

It is reasonably obvious that most of the physicians who practiced in Arkansas in the first half of the 19th century leaned toward the anti-contagionists viewpoint.

As to the illnesses they faced, we have an excellent source that fully documents the problems of disease in Arkansas. Dr. A. W. Webb lived and practiced in Chicot County in the 1840s. During his time he wrote a medical treatise on all of the illnesses he faced. The book is 700 pages, written in long hand and called *Medical Notes and Reflections*.

The list of aliments he enumerates is long and reflects many of the common maladies we see today. He talks very little of the chronic diseases of aging such as diabetes, heart disease and cancer. Since most of these illnesses only become obvious at an older age and long life was the exception in his day, this makes sense. He writes at length about problems of pregnancy and childbirth. The stethoscope had been invented in 1816 and he mentions its use. There are extended discussions of dyspepsia (peptic ulcer disease), traumatic diseases such as fractures and concussions, hysteria and insanity. Consumption and scrofula (two manifestations of tuberculosis) are discussed at length—the prevailing theory was that TB was a typical respiratory illness gone untreated; that if allowed to smolder it eventually consumed the system. He talks at length about the various infectious diseases such as smallpox, typhoid, measles, diphtheria, erysipelas, cholera, yellow fever and the various fevers. At one point he touches on the prevalent theories of miasma and epidemic constitution. In his words, "It is evident that, at times, certain atmospheric conditions, contain exhalations from the soil and certain electrical states concur and form an epidemic constitution through which agency a morbid poison propagates itself with unusual rapidity and intensity. The disease may be common marsh fever, yellow fever, bubo-plague or cholera depending on the circumstance of locality and habitat."

The majority of his text is spent detailing the various forms of fever: chief among them was Intermittent, Remittent and Bilious fevers. Most of these fevers, also called ague, were various forms of malaria. It would be another 70 years before the real culprits, the disease-carrying mosquito and the microorganism, Plasmodium, were identified and progress made toward eliminating this from the environs of Arkansas.

Malaria begins with a bite from an infected female mosquito; the plasmodium enters the circulation and ultimately the liver of the person; there it matures and reproduces. As the disease progresses there are high fevers and severe headaches. Depending on the variety of malaria the disease can result in coma and death or as is most often the case a recurring debilitating illness that may last for years. The various fevers and consumption regularly killed and debilitated large number of people but this was simply part of living in the Territory. The expectation was that when a person moved to Arkansas they would be sick for the first year or two, and if it did not kill them, they would be OK; the process was called seasoning. Much of the correspondence between those who lived in Arkansas and their families back east were framed around health. Often the letters began with: "I hope this note finds you well." Letters of the day are replete with references to "summer time illness" referring to fevers. "Like everyone here I suffer from the summer maladies. To this point I have not had to consult the doctor."

As with most physicians of his day Dr. Webb's heroic therapies involved mercury and antimony-based medicines, bleeding, induced vomiting or diarrhea and blistering on various parts of the body to rid it of the toxins; in hindsight the treatment was worse than the disease.

Mothers dying in childbirth and small children falling prey to first one illness and then another was common and an accepted part of life. Many of the young women who lived in Arkansas came from extended families that had provided health support and knowledge. In the new territory they were isolated and on their own. Pregnancy brought with it a number of unanswerable fears and concerns. Assuming the mother and baby survived the process of birth, the child was often not given a name at first. Only when the infant had shown itself to be strong enough to survive was it given a name.

Medical self-help books were important in day-to-day life in the country. Among these were Dr. Gunn's *Domestic Companion*, Thomason's *New Guide to Health*, Jonas Rishel's *The Indian Physician*, *A new system of Practice founded on Medicinal Plants*, and, later, R.V. Pierce's book, *The People's Common Sense Medical Advisor*. When a member of the family or a slave became ill, those who were literate consulted their book of choice or consulted with a neighbor who was literate. If their efforts failed and the illness persisted, they sent a runner for the doctor.

After the 1810s, increasing numbers of people who called themselves doctor moved into the state; most were based in the small towns and rode a circuit through the country. Generally, these physicians were trained in the European style of medicine and practiced the heroic forms of therapy like Dr. Webb. Their medical bag tended to be packed with many small bottles of basics which they compounded on site. They had a tendency to use significant amounts of mercury and antimony to the detriment of the patient. As with the American Indian medicine men they were good at external disease such as lancing boils, rashes and closed fractures. They did a reasonable job with childbirth when they were not forced to intervene. If they happened to be a "modern" and felt the need to intervene in childbirth, puerperal fever and death was often the case for the female.

There were generally two types of the European-trained physicians. The first were the university-trained physicians; they tended to look down on all other practitioners as quacks and charlatans. The second and, by far the majority, were the apprentice physicians who spent a specified time with a practicing physician, attended a period of two to three months at a proprietary medical school for additional training and then hung out his shingle.

In 1807 Samuel Hahnemann coined the phrase homeopathy as a reaction to the heroic measures of his day. The homeopathic physicians were similar to the European-trained physicians, but their doses of medicine were much more dilute, and they tended to stay away from heroic intervention and bleeding as forms of therapy. They focused on herbal medicines and to their credit less on heavy metals. Their long-term results were no better than that of the European-trained physicians, but at least they didn't make the patient sicker.

Midwives were often the most valuable resource for the community, and in the African-American communities they were often the only physician they knew. These women were trained in the techniques of childbirth by older midwives called Granny Midwives. Vestiges of this system were still in play in the middle of the 20th century. Because of their lack of information about the transmission of disease, their incidence of infection and death during childbirth was reasonably high.

Indian Medicine and Botanical doctors, the Patent Medicine doctors and Medicine Shows advertised regularly in the local papers. The Indian Medicine doctors would often claim to have received their knowledge directly from an old Indian while being held captive. Their medicines seldom had anything to do with the botanicals the Indians used and were more often than not a concoction of rum and syrup. Patent Medicine doctors had their special brand of secret cure, but only they knew the recipe. Medicine Shows were essentially a combination of Indian Medicine and Patent Medicine along with a good deal of entertainment.

In the mid-19th century, the Eclectic School of Medicine arrived, and as you might guess from the name, it was an amalgamation of all the various

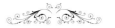

Letters in 19th century Arkansas were often focused on health: "I hope this note finds you well." Letters of that day are replete with references to "summer time illness" referring to fevers. "Like everyone here I suffer from the summer maladies. To this point I have not had to consult the doctor."

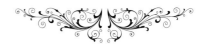

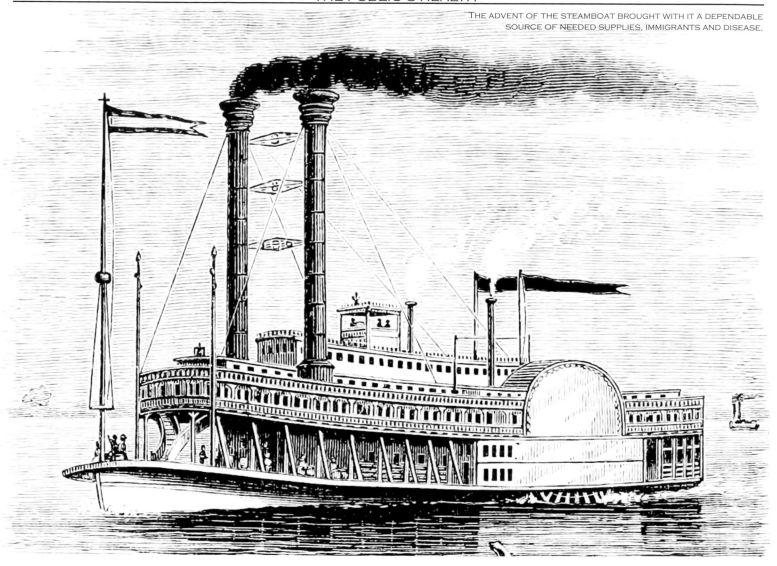

THE ADVENT OF THE STEAMBOAT BROUGHT WITH IT A DEPENDABLE
SOURCE OF NEEDED SUPPLIES, IMMIGRANTS AND DISEASE.

schools. In truth all of the men and women who practiced the trade of medicine were eclectic to some extent. The realities of daily life and the illnesses they faced made them look to anything that would help.

THE STEAMBOAT IS COMING

On April 20, 1820 the steamboat, Comet, made its way up the Arkansas River to Arkansas Post and ushered in a new era. Two years later, the Eagle made its way up river to Little Rock. In the next 10 years shallow-hulled steamboats made their way up the White, Black, Current and Little Red Rivers, parts of the St. Francis River, the Arkansas River to Fort Smith and the Ouachita River up to Camden. The Red River was slow in opening because of the great log jam that blocked the river in northwest Louisiana. Given the right water condition these boats provided a more reliable source of food commodities and necessary supplies. When the boats turned and made their way back downstream they carried with them the locally grown cotton and corn products to the wider world. Along with new immigrants, supplies and commerce these boats brought disease. The diseases that plagued the East Coast and New Orleans slowly began to make their way up the rivers and into the towns. As early as 1822, newspaper reports began to appear in the *Arkansas Gazette* of yellow fever on the Mississippi River as far north as Natchez, Mississippi.

Despite the fact that physicians of that time labored under faulty systems of diagnosis and treatment, there is little question that most of these men, even those with minimal training, were bright, literate, devoted to their patients and deeply involved in their communities. Though the general public had doubts about physicians as a whole, they valued and trusted their own doctor.

The first two communities to document the presence of physicians were Hix Ferry and Arkansas Post.

Hix Ferry was a river crossing on the Current River as the Southwest Trail entered Arkansas from Missouri. The ferry called the Gateway to Arkansas had been established by William Hix Sr. in 1801. Sometime early in the second decade of the 19th century, Dr. Peyton Pitman purchased the ferry from Mr. Hix. In addition to his duties as ferry operator and physician he also served as a Justice of the Peace, Judge in the Court of Common Complaints and the first Postmaster in the community of Fouche De Thomas. This tradition of physicians holding down a number of governmental positions continued throughout the nineteenth century.

At Arkansas Post the first to be mentioned is Dr. Robert F. Slaughter. The first mention of Dr. Slaughter is in 1812 when he was issued a license to engage in mercantile business at Arkansas Post in the district of Arkansas (it later became Arkansas County). Dr. Slaughter was apparently a wealthy man who owned a large amount of land along the Arkansas River.

It is clear that where one or more people congregated, a physician soon followed. By 1850 Arkansas had a population of 210,000 with 449 physicians and in 1860 the population had grown to 436,000 with 1,222 physicians. With the explosion in population, the towns and communities of Arkansas began to experience the various problems related to health and disease that the eastern cities and the Gulf Coast had dealt with since the 18th century.

While this growing population and their physicians labored away in relative obscurity on the frontier of the United States, they were in no way completely isolated. In 1819, William Woodruff founded the *Arkansas Gazette* at Arkansas Post and in late 1820 moved his newspaper to the tiny village of Little Rock. Little Rock was soon named the administrative center of the state. It was not the population center, that crown went to Lawrence County, the north central section of the territory centered on Batesville. In the early 1820s, 69 percent of the population lived along the Southwest Trail in that part of the territory. Little Rock was not the business center of the state; that fell first to northeast Arkansas because of the influx of population along the Southwest Trail. With the Indian removal of the late 1820s and 1830s, Fort Smith and Van Buren carried that mantle, and by the 1840s and 1850s, cotton, slavery and the large landowners of southeast Arkansas ruled the day.

With the production of a regular local newspaper, statewide, national and international news (albeit delayed sometimes by many months) became a part of the life of those who could read or knew someone who could read. As noted earlier, the arrival of the steamboat in the early 1820s made this transfer of information much easier.

Despite its isolation Arkansas was affected by a number of major events and changes that were going on beyond its borders. Europe, England and the eastern portion of the United States were constantly under the gun responding to one major epidemic after another. It was these responses that resulted in what we know as the modern Sanitation Movement of the 19th century and the beginnings of Public Health.

One area that was especially relevant to Arkansas was the development of several medical schools on the east coast. A number of the early physicians in Arkansas trained at the University of Pennsylvania, Columbia or Dartmouth before moving to Arkansas. Dr. Benjamin Rush, the head of the University of Pennsylvania, was one of the preeminent physicians in Colonial America. He was the chairman of medicine at the school, had an interest in use of botanical simples as medicine, the epidemics especially yellow fever and smallpox and the role of sanitation in preventing disease. Dr. Rush was a signatory of the Declaration of Independence and a good friend of Jefferson and Washington. During the Revolutionary War he was the Surgeon General for the Continental Army. During the exploration of the Louisiana Purchase all of the exploring parties were asked by Rush and Jefferson to comment on the state of health among the American Indians, the maladies from which they suffered and the various botanical treatments and remedies they used. In that day graduates of the medical school were required to complete a doctoral thesis, during Dr. Rush's tenure a number of those papers were on botanical simples (as the plant sources were called) and the uses that had been found for them.

It was during this time that the modern Sanitation movement of the 19th century had its beginning. The major cities of the east coast of the United States and New Orleans were being forced to deal with the impact of large concentrations of humans in small areas. The importance of clean water, disposal of sewage and waste and adequate housing became of paramount importance. Boston, New York City, Philadelphia, Savannah and New Orleans were faced with mammoth problems.

As their populations grew, each of the East Coast cities soon out stripped their clean water supplies. At this point in the history of the New World, local governments were not equipped to deal with problems such as animals and animal waste in the streets of the cities and the disposal of human waste. Most did not have sewer systems and any creek or stream soon became an open sewer. Following the lead of Europe and England, sanitation became a part of the social contract, cities and towns began to develop supplies of clean water, sewer systems were dug and scavengers were hired to clean the streets.

Much of what they were doing was re-creating the wheel. There is excellent evidence that the earliest civilizations in India, Mesopotamia, Egypt, Greece and Rome were knowledgeable about the needs of sanitation. There is good evidence of piped water and aqueducts designed to carry fresh water long distances, indoor flush toilets and covered sewer systems.

In 1819, a young man named Dr. Matthew Cunningham arrived in the small settlement of Little Rock. A native of Philadelphia, he had attended the

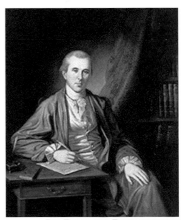

DR. BENJAMIN RUSH WAS THE DEAN OF AMERICAN MEDICINE AT THE TURN OF THE 19TH CENTURY. A COMTEMPORARY OF GEORGE WASHINGTON AND THOMAS JEFFERSON, HE TRAINED DR. MATTHEW CUNNINGHAM, THE FIRST FORMALLY TRAINED PHYSICIAN IN CENTRAL ARKANSAS.

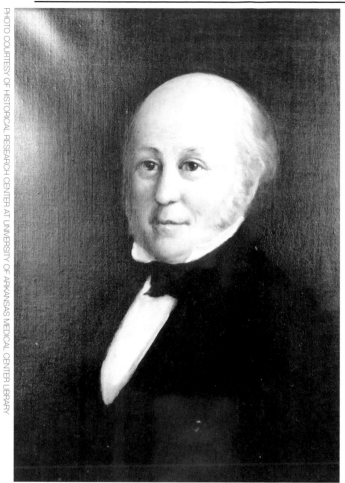

DR. MATTHEW CUNNINGHAM, THE FATHER OF MODERN MEDICINE IN CENTRAL ARKANSAS, THE FIRST MAYOR OF LITTLE ROCK, HELPED TO CREATE THE FIRST BOARD OF HEALTH.

University of Philadelphia Medical School under the tutelage of Dr. Benjamin Rush. After medical school he spent a brief time in Europe "seeking to improve himself in the practice of his profession." He first practiced in New Orleans for two years before returning to New York. In 1817 he moved with his wife to Missouri and two years later to Arkansas, leaving his wife in Missouri. It is alleged that he was the first permanent white European settler in Little Rock. Several notes indicate that when he arrived the only other building was a small shack used as a military post. Clearly, the American Indians had a presence in the area back as far as 1541; various travelers through the state mention homesteads up and down this part of the river. The probability is that Dr. Cunningham was one of the first settlers in Little Rock. His wife, followed him a year later, and she was most certainly the first white European female to call Little Rock home. Dr. Cunningham set up a practice, opened a pharmacy and became the Father of Modern Medicine in Central Arkansas. He was to be the first coroner, the first mayor of Little Rock and was instrumental in setting up the first Board of Health.

An interesting question that should be asked is: why Dr. Cunningham came all the way from the east coast to set up a practice of medicine and a pharmacy in a territory that had few people? Physicians, university-trained or not, weren't held in high esteem, and competition was stiff. There were no laws or regulations as to who could call themselves a doctor, and the general public did not differentiate between those with a degree and those without. Because of the large number of physicians, competition was stiff, and the first man to hang out a shingle had a leg up on the competition. A significant number of physicians saw themselves as only part-time doctors using medicine as a spring board into business or politics. Many of the physicians who populated the state went on to become prominent politicians in the state of Arkansas.

SMALLPOX

The winter of 1824 saw massive flooding along the White and the Mississippi Rivers followed by two extremely hot summers. There were several reports of unhealthy conditions of life in Arkansas and specifically Little Rock. Most of the illnesses and deaths appeared to have been one of a variety of fevers (malaria). In September 1825, there were reports of major illness and death among the Cherokee Indians at Dwight Mission in West Central Arkansas. In April 1826, there was a widespread outbreak of a flu-like illness in the Little Rock area.

In 1826, smallpox began to be reported along the middle Mississippi Valley. The disease is caused by the virus Variola Major and made its first appearance in human populations 2,500 to 3,000 years ago. There is evidence that it has decimated populations in India, Asia and North Africa with epidemics for at least three millennia. Though it was present in Southeastern Europe it did not have a major impact until the population began to increase at about the time of the Crusades.

The illness is transmitted by inhalation of the Variola virus usually through direct contact with an infected person, exposure to bodily fluids or contaminated objects such as blankets or clothing. From initial contact with the virus, it takes 10-12 days to develop the illness. It begins with a fever and flu-like symptoms, and two days later the person begins to breakout in widespread blisters that eventually have the appearance of pustules. As these blisters heal they form scabs and deep scars. If the blisters become confluent there is a 60 percent death rate. In the worse cases these lesions will become hemorrhagic.

The first documented outbreak of smallpox in Arkansas struck the small community of Arkansas Post on the Mississippi. The illness was purported to have been brought up river by steamboat from New Orleans where an epidemic was in process. By all appearances it did not make major inroads into the rest of the state; however, the fear of this disease was great. During this time several articles gave a blow-by-blow record of the illness and death that were occurring down river with the admonition that it was only a matter of time before it spread to the rest of the state.

Unlike most of the other illnesses that early Arkansans faced there was an effective remedy for smallpox. Since 1000 B.C.E. the process of variolation had been used in the Far East. With variolation, the dried matter of smallpox scabs were inserted into the nose or into a broken area of skin. It was effective in creating immunity but often caused active smallpox. Lady Mary Worthy Montague brought the process to England in 1718 and promoted it. In 1796

Dr. Edward Jenner, a doctor in rural England, who was aware of the process of variolation, discovered that immunity to smallpox could be achieved by inoculating individuals with material from a cowpox lesion. The cowpox virus is similar to the smallpox but does not infect humans. He termed the material used for inoculation, vaccine (from the root word vacca, Latin for cow). Eventually the cox pox virus was replaced by the vaccine virus, a similar family to cowpox and smallpox. Soon after his discovery the smallpox vaccination was being used all over the world. On March 21, 1826, the editor of the *Gazette* admonished and pleaded with its readers to have the smallpox vaccination or Kine Pox matter. He went on to say that Dr. Cunningham had fresh vaccine matter that he had just received from Nashville by the last mail.

The first real foray into the public's health in Arkansas was an ordinance passed in the town of Little Rock on July 1, 1826. The title of the ordinance was Removal of Nuisances. "That any dead horse, cow, hog or any other animal found lying on any of the streets of said town, it will be the duty of the constable to have such animals removed, for which services he will receive fifty cents." The ordinance goes on to talk about dead animals on private properties that are a nuisance and their removal. If one looks at the patterns of development of larger communities most of the towns and cities along the east coast had passed similar scavenger ordinances during the eighteenth century at the same point in their development

At the end of the 1820s Arkansas had doubled its population to 30,000 and by 1840 the population tripled to 100,000. The 1830s saw the removal of American Indians from the state increasing the importance of Fort Smith and Van Buren from an economic and health standpoint. At the same time the delta lands began to open up, and the slave population began to grow.

In 1831, another outbreak of smallpox occurred, and this time it didn't stop at the mouth of the Arkansas River. It appeared first in February with the arrival of the steamboat, Waverly, in Little Rock from Natchez. An African-American male on board the ship became ill soon after arriving at Little Rock. It quickly became apparent that he had smallpox and as the editor of the paper wrote, "the proper authorities removed the infected individual to a place where he could be taken care of, without endangering the safety and lives of our citizens." The gentleman did die and for a week or two Little Rock business boosters took control, casting question as to whether he really had smallpox or something else less virulent. This tactic had been and continued to be common throughout the 19th and early 20th century. The obvious reasoning was that a virulent epidemic disease left the wrong impression with outsiders and hurt business. Their ruse might have worked except for the fact that several other cases developed in the next few weeks. During that year other cases of smallpox were reported in Arkansas Post, Chicot and Phillips counties. For the next 70 years, the people of Arkansas were plagued with recurring rounds of smallpox.

In 1831, the territorial legislature passed a Medical Licensing Bill. This bill written by the university-trained physicians of the state specified the requirements for licensing and practice of medicine. The bill required the establishment of a self-perpetuating board of eight learned physicians (read: university-trained) who examined all candidates who wished to practice medicine or surgery. If the physician had a university degree, he did not have to be examined. Upon passing the exam the physician was required to pay a $15 fee. Anyone caught practicing without a license was fined $200-$500 for the first offense, double that fine for a second offense with six months in jail; there was no appeal from the board. This measure was a pretty open power play to eliminate their competition. An additional motive behind the bill was to assure that the duly licensed physician could collect his fees in court. Despite the fact that the bill was passed, Territorial Governor Pope vetoed the bill. As an appointee of Andrew Jackson and a staunch populist he was not about to see the establishment of "an intellectual aristocracy in this remote place." He went on to say that "physicians, who have been in full and successful practice for many years and had received a diploma from the highest authority in the land, public opinion, are prohibited from pursing their profession until they pay their fifteen dollars, and obtain a license from this Board."

The first U. S. physician licensing law was passed in Massachusetts in 1819; almost all of the states eventually did the same. In most cases, just as in Arkansas, the laws were vetoed, repealed within a year or two or modified to the point that they were powerless. By 1850, only Louisiana, Michigan, New Jersey and

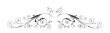

Territorial Governor Pope vetoed the bill for medical licenses. As an appointee of Andrew Jackson and a staunch populist he was not about to see the establishment of "an intellectual aristocracy in this remote place." He went on to say that "physicians, who have been in full and successful practice for many years and had received a diploma from the highest authority in the land, public opinion, are prohibited from pursing their profession until they pay their fifteen dollars, and obtain a license from this Board."

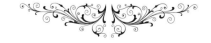

Washington, D.C. had laws concerning the licensing of physicians.

Indian removal, cholera and public health

The 1830s were a time of great flux; the population increased dramatically and the quest for statehood was fulfilled in 1836. The defining set of events in the health of Arkansas revolved around the Choctaw Indian Removal and the emergence of cholera.

The removal of the Choctaws of Mississippi to Oklahoma took place over a three year timeframe, 1831 to 1833. In October 1831, the Choctaws to be moved were allowed two weeks to gather their crops, assemble their personal property and sell their homes. They were divided into two groups; the first group was to ferry across the river at Memphis and take the northern route up the Arkansas River, and the second was to meet at Vicksburg and then be moved up the Red and Ouachita Rivers to John Camden's Post (Camden) and from there hauled over land to Fort Towson in south east Oklahoma. By late October large encampments sprang up around the outskirts of Memphis and Vicksburg; and then it began to rain. Soon the river bottomlands of the Mississippi, Arkansas and Ouachita Rivers were flooded making the removal by wagons impossible. The removal agents realized they had no other option but to round up all available steamboats and take the river route. In mid-November 2,000 Choctaws were crammed onto the Walter Scott and the Reindeer. At Arkansas Post the U.S. Army forced the Choctaw to leave the boats and commandeered the boats for use in troop transport. Following the floods, a blizzard struck the poorly provisioned Choctaws and within a few days all of the provisions were gone. They were reduced to a ration of a handful of parched corn, one turnip and two cups of heated water a day. Below freezing temperature continued for eight days, and the steamboats could not make it back down stream to pick up the Choctaws. Eight days later, a train of wagons and supplies arrived from Little Rock. When the Choctaw finally arrived in Little Rock one of the chiefs, Thomas Harkins, in an interview with the *Arkansas Gazette*, remarked that so far the removal had been "a trail of tears and death." Many of the Choctaw had frozen to death or died of pneumonia. The 3,000 Choctaws who were taken the southern route did not fare any better. The guides who were leading them to Oklahoma got lost in the swamps around Lake Providence, Louisiana. They ultimately made it to Camden but by that time they were plagued by dysentery, diphtheria and typhoid.

The estimates are that of the 6,000 total that left for Oklahoma in that first year only 4,000 made it to their new homes.

Logically the southern route, even though it had its own problems, should have been the reasonable choice for the second year of removal, but that was not to be. The plan was for all of the Choctaws to be gathered at Vicksburg, transported by boat to Arkansas Post and then marched across the East Arkansas delta swamps. The Choctaws began gathering at Vicksburg in early October. As they were gathering, an epidemic of cholera broke out. Cholera had raged in Europe for several years and in the summer of 1832 made its first appearance in Montreal, Canada. By the fall it had made its way to New Orleans.

Like smallpox, cholera struck fear in the hearts of the population. It is an infection of the bowel caused by the bacteria Vibrio cholerae. The main symptoms are an overwhelming profuse, watery diarrhea and vomiting that quickly lead to dehydration and death. Infection occurs through the drinking or eating of food or water that has been contaminated by the feces of an infected person, often someone with no symptoms.

When word of cholera among the Indians reached the residents of Vicksburg they quickly abandoned the town for the countryside taking the disease with them. Most of those who became ill, Choctaw and white European alike, died, and soon bodies were heaped into piles, covered with brush and burned.

One thousand of the Choctaws who had not made it to Vicksburg were diverted to Memphis where they boarded a commandeered snag boat, the Archimedes. They were taken to Arkansas Post, met by government wagons and taken by land to Little Rock and on to Oklahoma. The remnants of the Choctaws left in Vicksburg were brought upriver on the Brandywine, but by the time they arrived the rains had begun again. The decision was made to take them up the White River to Rock Row (near present day Clarendon). Here the cholera struck again with a vengeance. It eventually subsided, but again there was a significant loss of life.

There were no accurate figures kept of how many Choctaw began the trips in 1831 and 1832, but estimates are that there were 7,000-9,000. Deaths for the first two years of the removal probably amounted to somewhere in the range of 3,000 or a fourth of the population of the Choctaw from Mississippi.

As cholera epidemics spread across North America, temporary Boards of Health were set up in each of the major cities and were effective to some extent in quarantining some of the disease.

The city fathers of Little Rock followed this disease as it progressed across the country. On November 3, 1832, the Town Council, with Dr. Cunningham as mayor, passed a resolution appointing a Board of Health. The board consisted of William Stevenson as president and William Woodruff as secretary. Also on the board were Doctors M. Cunningham, B.W. Lee, Alden Sprague and R. A. Watkins. These men were charged with making arrangements for the erection of a temporary building to be used as a hospital for all strangers and indigent people laboring under the cholera or any infectious or other contagious disease demanding the care and attention of the Board. The doctors on the Board of Health formed a committee to draft an address to the community admonishing them on the danger to which they would be exposed in the event of cholera in the community and advising them on the steps to prevent spreading of the disease. Stevenson and Woodruff were appointed to a committee to visit the premises of several rooming houses in the town for the purpose of ascertaining if any nuisances about them could be calculated to generate disease and endanger the health of the citizens. The board was to contact Capt. Brown, Disbursing Agent for the Choctaw Removal, and respectfully request that he choose a convenient route through Central Arkansas that did not involve the streets of Little Rock. An additional request was that he prevent straggling parties of Indians from wandering the streets of Little Rock. The goals of the board were quarantine, education and sanitation.

This date and this meeting should probably go down in history as the real beginning of public health in Arkansas.

The board rented a house from Mr. N. W. Maynor situated about a mile west of town to be used as a Cholera Hospital. It was resolved that it would be the duty of the medical members of the board to board any ship or other conveyance and report any infectious disease.

When the board received word that cholera had broken out among the Choctaw at Rock Roe, they dispatched Dr. B.W. Lee to Rock Roe to consult with the physicians who were working among the Choctaw and report back to the board. In four days, they received a letter from Dr. Lee indicating that at the height of the epidemic there were as many as 16 deaths a day. He suggested that the disease may have been caused by the overcrowding on the steamboats and a sudden change in diet. This is the first piece of public health investigation of a disease outbreak in Arkansas.

There was another article several days later indicating the Capt. Brown had taken prompt action to prevent the Indians from coming through the streets of town.

An article appeared in the paper on Nov. 12 with the headline: TO THE CITIZENS OF LITTLE ROCK. This article outlined the steps that could be taken by the average citizen to avoid the disease, and the most important points were: cleanliness, avoid excessive fatigue and exposure to damp chills of evening air.

Near the end of the article it states, "This epidemic is confidently affirmed not to be contagious in its character." It would be another 20 years before John Snow, the British researcher and investigator, showed that the disease was in fact contagious; it was in the water.

By 1840 the Arkansas population had grown to 98,000, in 1850 to 210,000 and in 1860 to 436,000. With this doubling of population every 10 years reports of epidemics and mini-epidemics became common place.

Throughout the 1830s, epidemics of cholera, flu, typhoid and smallpox were reported yearly. Between 1848 and 1851, cholera hit with a vengeance striking communities of all sizes along the waterways of Arkansas. During the 1840s and 1850s, scarlet fever and the flu were reported with increased frequency. In 1855 the state had its first documented taste of yellow fever in the towns of Napoleon and Helena on the Mississippi River.

As the population grew, local papers, community groups and politicians increasingly turned their attention to issues related to public health. In 1838, a Little Rock ordinance was passed that required all steamboats approaching the city closer than one-quarter mile be inspected by a physician checking the passengers for signs of cholera, smallpox and other contagious disease.

The town of Little Rock was bisected by a small stream called the Town Branch. It began in the area of what would be present day south Louisiana Street, made a loop toward the river and then turned southeast eventually emptying into Fouche Creek. With no system dealing with waste, Town Branch became an open sewer. Dead animals, overflow from privies and the remains of chamber pots were dumped into Town Branch. Since it was a meandering stream clogged with trees and human debris the least rain resulted in flooding. Mayor Cunningham proposed that the branch be turned into a canal to make sure that it drained. This would be the first of many proposals and projects relating to Town Branch for the next half century. The problem was not solved until Little Rock had an adequate sewer system.

In 1840, an ordinance was passed authorizing the shooting of hogs running loose in the streets. In January 1841, slaughterhouses and the hawking of wild game were banned from the city.

In the mid-1840s, there were complaints of raw sewage and fowl smelling pools of stagnant water in the streets of downtown Little Rock. During

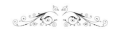

Statement in the newspaper regarding cholera: "This epidemic is confidently affirmed not to be contagious in its character."

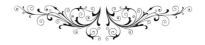

times of threatened disease outbreaks, the city council created temporary boards of health and made an effort at cleaning up the city. They aggressively pursued any nuisances they thought might create an epidemic constitution for disease. One of the common techniques was to remove the offending decaying material and use a liberal amount of lime. Once the crisis had passed the temporary boards were dissolved.

In the 1850s, water became an important issue in any town of size. By 1859, the town of Little Rock had grown to 6,000 and the threat of fire was an increasing problem. In addition to the fire hazard, drinking water supplies were becoming unreliable especially during seasons of drought. It was proposed that the city bore an artesian well on some prominent eminence. Similar proposals were made for the towns of Monticello, Des Arc and Crossett.

As with public health measures, the increase in population helped to develop constituencies for other health related activities. As early as 1850, a Reverend Chaplin of Fort Smith started classes for blind readers and was soliciting aid for rehabilitation of the blind. In 1851, the Clarksville Institute announced that they would be teaching free classes for deaf mutes. In 1854 there was an attempt to develop a poor house for the destitute in Little Rock. In December 1851, the first hospital in Arkansas was opened in Napoleon, Arkansas. There had been several sick houses during times of epidemics but this was the first facility built for the designed purpose of being a hospital. It and three other hospitals were built along the Mississippi by the U.S. Marine Corps to deal with sick seaman, pilots and engineers who worked up and down the river.

During the late 1850s, a number of proposals for worthwhile projects were discussed in the local paper such as the formation of a medical school, the building of an insane asylum and the establishment of a medical society. These worthwhile projects would have to wait; the country had a war to fight.

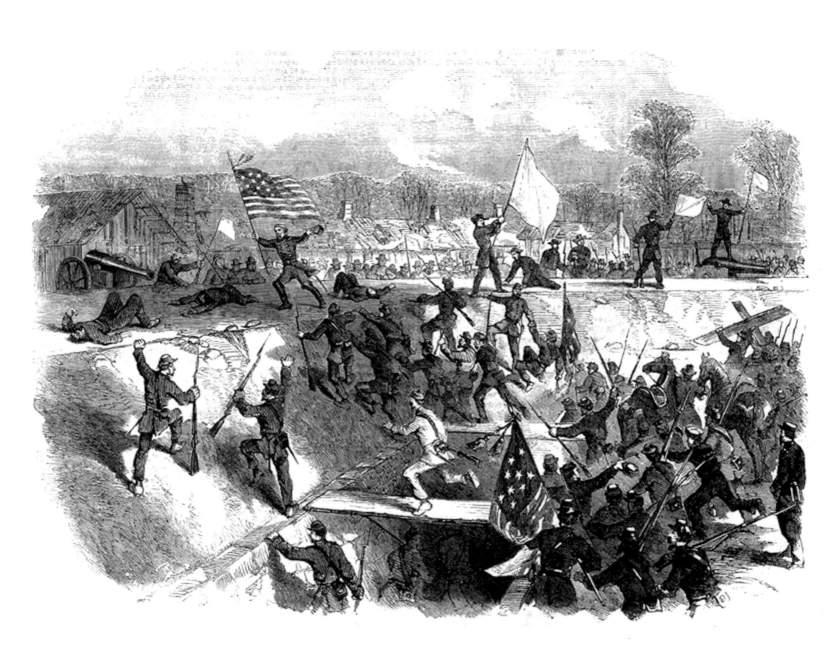

Disease, famine, wound infection and illness accounted for far more deaths during the Civil War than the immediate effect of gunshot wounds.

CHAPTER FOUR
THE CIVIL WAR AND ITS AFTERMATH

The second half of the 19th century was a time of major change in the life of the people of Arkansas: first the Civil War, then Reconstruction and the Financial Panic of 1873 followed by the Long Depression and finally the Panic and Depression of 1893. It wasn't until the first decade of the 20th century that Arkansas began to make progressive changes with an eye toward prosperity.

The population grew from 436,000 in 1860 to 1.6 million in 1910; the cities of Arkansas grew as well—Pine Buff had grown to a population of 15,000, Fort Smith to 24,000 and Little Rock/North Little Rock was at 57,000. Even with the growth of these towns, 87 percent of the population lived in a rural setting.

Many of the changes that ultimately affected health and disease in Arkansas had their origin far beyond the borders of the state. The proliferation of railroads in the post war era created new towns and caused others to fade away. The demand for timber products triggered a new export industry and resulted in a major influx of immigrants. An insatiable need for energy caused a coal mining boom in the Arkansas River Valley. Changes in medicine and the understanding of health and disease revolutionized life during this time.

THE GERM THEORY EMERGES

The changes in the understanding of disease had been coming for at least 200 years. Thomas Sydenham (1624-1689) developed the concept of disease as an entity, an objective thing in itself that could be observed, described and classified; he contended that disease was separate from the various symptoms it caused. Needless to say his ideas fought a losing battle against the established Humeral Theory of Health and Disease until the middle of the 19th century.

By the middle of the 19th century there was a consilience of ideas that resulted in a major shift in how health and disease were viewed. In Vienna in 1847, Ignaz Semmelwesis demonstrated that postpartum fever and infection could be reduced to less than one percent with the simple washing of hands when going from patient to patient. At first he was laughed at and ignored, but his ideas were eventually validated. John Snow in England did groundbreaking work in 1854 in London during a cholera outbreak when he discovered that the source of the disease was a hand pump that had been contaminated by a faulty sewer. In the late 1850s, Louis Pasteur in France got much of the credit for formulating the germ theory. In fairness this idea had been around for a long time but he was one of the first to demonstrate the validity of the idea and convince the powerful forces of science and medicine. In 1865, Dr. Joseph Lister, an English surgeon, put the germ theory to a practical test. He demonstrated that the use of antisepsis (a surgeon washing his hands before surgery and cleaning the wound with carbolic acid) reduced the risk of surgical infection as much

An equally important area of advance was the development of what was first called political arithmetic, and what we now call vital statistics; an accurate accounting of life, death and the various factors that affect human existence. As with the medical side of the equation the changes began as early as the mid-17th century. One of the first and most important lessons learned was the "negative urban penalty"—that people who lived in industrialized cities, in crowded substandard housing with inadequate clean water and no sewage system had a higher risk of premature death and disease and a disproportion of this premature death fell on infants. By the mid-19th century, it became quite obvious that accurate data about health and disease were essential if any headway was to be made in the forms of pestilence that human populations dealt with. In 1871, Dr. Roscoe Green Jennings was instrumental in establishing the first vital statistics ordinance in Little Rock.

In the early 21st century the information float time—the time it takes for something to be discovered, verified and disseminated to rest of the world—is often measured in terms of weeks or months. In the 19th century, the information float time was measured in decades. The events described above took several generations to be fully implemented and none would be accepted and in common use during the Civil War.

SLAVERY, THE CIVIL WAR AND DISEASE IN ARKANSAS

In 1804, there were no more than 60 black slaves in Arkansas. By 1860, there was a total population of 436,000 and 111,000 were black slaves. They were not evenly distributed across the state; the majority was in the southeast and south central part of the state. At the beginning of the Civil War, 81 percent of the population in Chicot county were black slaves; they were the economic foundation on which the antebellum mansion of King Cotton was built. Because of their importance in the industry, a good deal is known about their illnesses and the effect it had on productivity. Before the Civil War, a young black man free of disease was worth $1,000 but one with any sign of disease was valued at no greater than $500. A young black woman provided value in two ways, first as a worker and second as a source of babies and new slaves. There is recorded the case of Sevella, a 22-year-old black slave who had scrofula (tuberculosis), being worth $500 as opposed to other young women of her age who were valued at $1,200.

The range of illnesses that affected the slave population was similar to that of the white European population. Malaria (by a variety of names) was most common. Cholera was a major killer in the late 1840s and early 1850s. Scarlet fever, croup, eye diseases, whooping cough, measles, convulsions, dysentery, and meningitis were commonly reported. In the adult populations, gonorrhea and syphilis were a frequent complaint. Among the slave children, scarlet fever, croup and dysentery were common causes of death. On a per-capita basis, cholera and whooping cough were far more likely to result in death to a black slave than to a white. Malaria and yellow fever, two illnesses of tropical origin, were less likely to result in death to the black slave. During the yellow fever outbreaks of the second half of the 19th century, freedmen were often recruited as nurses.

With the Civil War and the Emancipation Proclamation in 1863, the

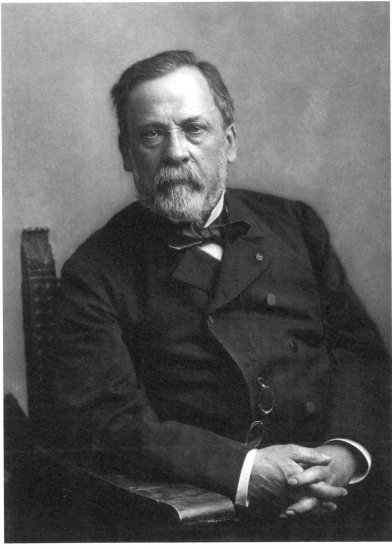

BEST KNOWN FOR THE PROCESS OF PASTEURIZATION OF MILK AND WINE, BUT MORE IMPORTANTLY, LOUIS PASTEUR CONVINCED MAIN-STREAM SCIENCE OF THE VALIDITY OF THE GERM THEORY.

as 80 percent. In the early 1870s, Dr. Robert Koch discovered that anthrax in cows was caused by a microscopic rod-shaped organism and could be passed from cow to cow. Using the same scientific postulates he went on to identify the bacteria that caused tuberculosis. In a short span of time his students identified the organisms that caused diphtheria, typhoid, pneumonia, gonorrhea, meningitis, leprosy, bubonic plague, tetanus, and syphilis.

Along with the prevention of surgical wound infection, the advent of effective anesthesia in the form of nitrous oxide, ether and chloroform revolutionized surgery; antisepsis (cleanliness), hemostasis (preventing bleeding) and gentleness with tissue became the new rules of surgery.

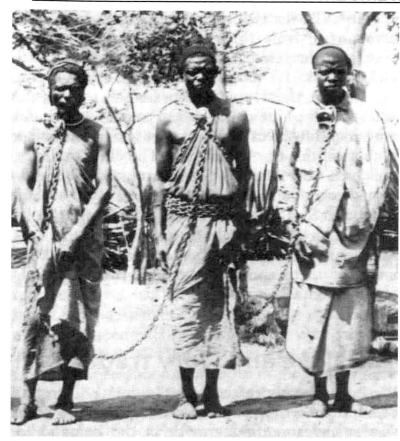

BLACK SLAVES CHAINED TOGETHER AT THE NECK.

111,000 people who had been held in slavery were now free. Since almost all of the war was fought on southern soil—crop production dropped to near zero, imported food stuffs were scarce, medicines were nonexistent, there was no one to work the fields and in many instances local government ceased to exist. Famine and epidemics were common.

Disease, famine, wound infection and illness accounted for far more deaths during the conflict than the immediate effect of a gunshot wound. The Confederate Army was composed mostly of conscripted soldiers who had never been more than a few miles from home and commanded by officers who had few qualifications had far more problems with sanitation issues and epidemic disease. Among the Federal troops there was a cadre of seasoned Regular Army commanders who understood, at least to some extent, the importance of sanitation, of clean water and sewage problems and general hygiene. The Sanitary Commission charged with dealing with sanitation and care and treatment of the injured soldiers was well aware of the problems but very little could be done. In the course of the war, smallpox played a significant role in several battles in Arkansas. A Confederate staging area at White Sulfur Springs, south of Pine Bluff, was struck with an outbreak of smallpox thought to have been brought in by volunteers from Texas. There were reports that the Battle of Brownsville in Lonoke County was affected by smallpox as well. The Federal troops stationed in Helena were plagued with the "Fever" to the point that less than half of the force could be mustered on any one day.

After 1863 and the Federal occupation of large segments of Arkansas, many of the newly freed slaves began to flood into the Federal camps. The troops and their commanders were trained to fight war and not to take care of civilians. By 1864 there were Freedmen Camps in Pine Bluff, Helena, Little Rock, Camden and DeValls Bluff. Eventually Fort Smith, Washington and Napoleon were added to this list. The Federal Freedman Bureau was created in 1865 and it was faced with monumental problems. Famine and disease were widespread. At Pine Bluff the main killers were measles, mumps, whooping cough, pneumonia and dysentery; over 10 percent of the camp died in the summer of 1864. Smallpox raged at DeValls Bluff. In the town of Osceola, 70 people died of cholera during the summer of 1866. Cholera struck the camp at Little Rock in August 1866 killing four Freedmen a day. In the summer of 1867, cholera struck in Fort Smith, Little Rock, Madison, Helena and Pine Bluff.

Medicine and doctors were scarce. Most towns in Arkansas refused to help the black Freedman. Despite the epidemics in their town, the city fathers of Helena refused to act on behalf of the black population. The Jacksonport mayor offered assistance to white paupers but not black. The Little Rock city fathers refused assistance toward the relief of the black refugees.

By 1867, the Freedman's Bureau established a number of facilities across the state that were designated as hospitals but it is important to remember that these were less like modern hospitals and more like poor houses. Most of these designated hospitals were filthy, with little or no equipment, no medicine and almost no staff.

Jefferson county, June 9, 1851.   6—5w.

Runaway Negro in Jail.

WAS committed to the Jail of Saline county, as a runaway, on the 8th day of June, 1851, a negro man, who says his name is JOHN, and that he belongs to *Henry Johnson*, of Desha county, Ark. He is aged about 24 or 25 years, straight in stature, quick spoken, looks very fierce out of his eyes, and plays on the fiddle. Had on, when apprehended, white cotton pants, coarse cotton shirt, and black hat. The owner is hereby notified to come forward, prove property, and pay the expenses of committal and advertisement, otherwise the said negro will be dealt with according to law.   THOMAS PACK, *Sheriff and Jailor of Saline county.*
Benton, June 21, 1851.   7—26w.

Pay up! Pay up!!

ALL persons indebted to the undersigned, whose notes and accounts are now due, are requested to call and pay up, by the 1st day of July next.   JOHN D. ADAMS.
June 13, 1851.   5—

Thirty Dollars Reward.

LEFT my plantation, in Arkansas county, near Post of Arkansas, on the 26th May (ult.), two Negro Men, viz:
GEORGE, a dark copper-colored man, about 30 years of age, 5 ft. 8 or 10 inches high, forehead rather low, some beard on his chin, stutters considerably and has a habit of winking his eyes when talking. He was recently purchased from Mr. Wm. E. Woodruff, at Little Rock, and has a wife at Dr. Watkins', near that city.
Also, HARRISON, about the same age, as the other, and belongs to Mr. W. R. Perry, of the same county.
The above slaves left in company, and it is supposed will make for Little Rock.
The above reward will be paid for arresting and securing said negroes, so that their owners may get them, or one-half the amount for either of them. Letters will reach me if addressed to Arkansas Post, Ark's.   J. FLOYD SMITH.
Arkansas co., June 6, 1851.   4—tf.

THE WHITE PHYSICIANS SUFFERED FROM A FORM OF "MORAL ASTIGMATISM." SLAVES WHO REPEATEDLY RAN AWAY WERE DIAGNOSED AS HAVING THE DISEASE DRAPETOMANIA.

As in earlier times of crisis, several temporary Boards of Health were established. In 1866, as a response to the cholera season, Little Rock created a Board of Health giving it the power to clean the streets and tear down facilities that were apparently hazardous to the public's health.

By 1867, the Freedman's Bureau lost most of its funding and all of the facilities in Arkansas were forced to close. A devil's bargain had been struck; slavery was gone but it was quickly replaced by sharecropping, peonage, the Ku Klux Klan and Jim Crow.

YELLOW FEVER

The year 1869 saw the completion of the Memphis to Little Rock railway. By 1872, the rail line running south from St. Louis was connected to Little Rock. As with the steamboats in the 1920s, the railroads reduced the isolation of Arkansas, dramatically increased migration and sped up the potential transmission of disease from one community to the next. It did not take long for this potential problem to be tested.

Cholera made its presence known in the Western Hemisphere in 1832 and for several decades was the most feared disease in the Mid-South; this crown was about to be handed off to yellow fever.

Yellow fever is a viral illness transmitted by the bite of the female Aedes aegypti mosquito. It is thought to have become endemic in the Western Hemisphere with the importation of black slaves from Africa. It hit first in the Caribbean and for a century and a half there were periodic epidemics on the East and Caribbean coastal cities of the United States. These epidemics continued to recur until a final scourge in New Orleans in 1905.

It is a frightful and violent illness that begins three to six days after the bite, initially presenting as a flu-like illness. Very often there is a brief period where the patient thinks they are recovering only to progress to the toxic phase of the illness with severe headache, dramatic recurring fevers, jaundice, massive gastrointestinal bleeding, liver and kidney failure. Of those who become toxic a high percentage die. In the 19th century there was no treatment except

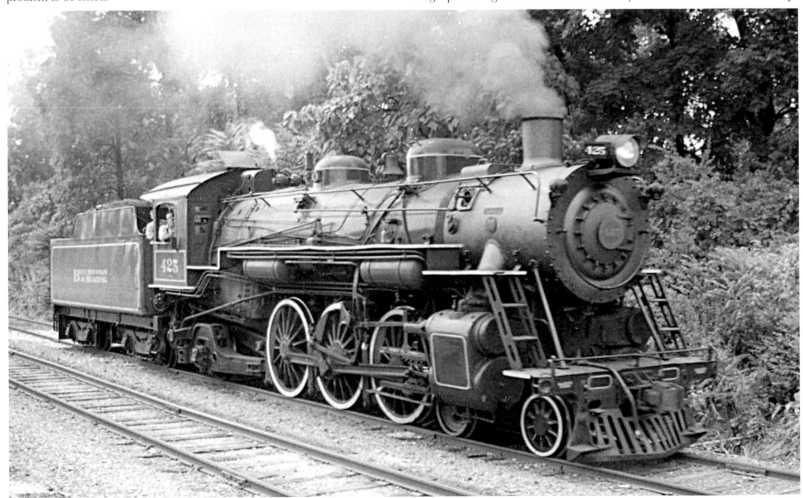

ARKANSAS DID NOT BENEFIT FROM THE GILDED AGE EXCEPT FOR THE BUILDING OF RAILROADS. THESE RAILROADS BROUGHT A BOOM IN THE POPULATION AND A MORE RAPID SPREAD OF DISEASE.

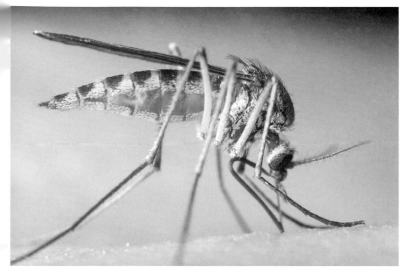

MALARIA AND YELLOW FEVER, TWO DISEASES OF AFRICAN ORIGIN TRANSMITTED MY MOSQUITOES, PLAYED A MAJOR ROLE IN THE LIFE OF 19TH AND EARLY 20TH CENTURY ARKANSAS.

supportive care. It wasn't until the 20th century and the understanding of the role of the mosquito in this illness that progress was made in dealing with yellow fever.

With the advent of the steamboat in the early 19th century, towns on the Mississippi had begun to experience epidemics of yellow fever. Probably because of the limited population of Arkansas it was spared until 1855. In that year yellow fever struck in Helena and Napoleon. Dr. Charles Edward Nash, a physician in Helena, wrote eloquently of the outbreak in his biographical sketches of Confederate Generals Pat Cleburne and General T. C. Hindman.

William Barnett, a young newspaper boy, boarded a docked steamer, which had just arrived in Helena from down river, to sell his newspapers. Unknown to the city fathers of the town the steamer carried passengers who were ill with yellow fever, several had already died. Since there had never been a case of yellow fever in Helena there was no Board of Health or any other precautions. In a short time the boy was ill, as were his two brothers and two sisters. Eventually one of his sisters died. Most of those who boarded the steamer became ill. As word spread, the citizens of Helena voted with their feet and abandoned the town, soon the town of 1,500 was reduced to a ghost town. Only a few people were left and it fell to them to minister to the sick and dying. Dr. Nash and two other physicians made their rounds daily and soon one of them was ill. Nash speaks in glowing terms of three men who helped him as nurses: Pat Cleburne, T. C. Hindman and a young minister named Rice. These three men agreed to cook, clean and perform nursing duties for the ill. The siege lasted for two months and when it was over many had died; there were no exact numbers. The young newsboy did survive and went on to be one of the leading journalists in the state. This same sequence of events had been playing out for at least a century in the United States but

these were the first documented cases in the state of Arkansas.

The city of Memphis was struck with yellow fever in 1828, 1855 and in 1867 but none of these outbreaks compared to the 1870s. The 1873 epidemic claimed 2,000 lives. Quickly after the fever hit, the citizens of Memphis began to flee in a wholesale fashion. Many used the trains and by September 18 it was obvious that many of the fleeing citizens were heading in the direction of Arkansas. Ultimately, there were several cases and at least three deaths reported in Argenta (North Little Rock). The temporary Health Board of Little Rock, with the acquiescence of the city government, imposed a quarantine aimed primarily at rail and steamboat travelling from Memphis and eventually included Argenta in this quarantine. In the end, there was at least one case in Little Rock and one in Pine Bluff, but by the time of the first frost most cases in the region had disappeared. During this same summer, Shreveport, Louisiana, a town of 4,000 people, lost 795 to yellow fever. It is important to remember that just because no disease or deaths were reported does not mean that none was there. Almost 90 percent of the citizens of the state lived on the farm and most in small family groups scattered across the state. There was clearly yellow fever up and down the Mississippi and Red River and it is highly probable that several of the small communities on the Arkansas side of the river were affected. With the first cold snap and the death of a large part of the mosquitoes the epidemic abated. It is fair to assume that the road and rail quarantine of traffic from Memphis spared Central Arkansas.

Even though the towns along the Mississippi were prepared for a repeat performance in 1874, it did not occur until 1878.

On August 1, 1878, William Warren, a steamboat crew member from a boat docked at Presidents Island, entered the city of Memphis. One day later he was admitted to the City Hospital and two days later he was dead. When word got out of a yellow fever death in the city, the citizens again began to flee. Schools and churches closed their doors. Passenger boat services from New Orleans were forced to disembark their passengers on the Arkansas side. The steamship John D. Porter took people fleeing Memphis northward in hopes of escaping the disease, but passengers were not allowed to disembark due to concerns of spreading yellow fever. The ship roamed the Mississippi River for the next two months before unloading its passengers. Seven thousand people died in the city of Memphis. This would be the last straw for the city; it was unincorporated and taken over by the state of Tennessee for a period of time.

When they heard of the yellow fever, the temporary Little Rock Board of Health composed of businessmen and physicians began making preparations. Convict labor was used to begin cleaning the streets and eliminating hazards to the public's health. A number of quarantines of rail, steamboat and wagon were established. Technically, the Board of Health in Little Rock had no jurisdiction five miles beyond the border of the city. At first this did not seem to concern the general populace. The major objections to the arbitrary "illegal" quarantine were by the businessmen who depended on the trains for business. For several weeks, there was a rather heated debate about the wisdom of the quarantine. The physicians of the community and businessmen on the board could not agree as to the right course to take. In the end the citizens of Little Rock demanded the quarantine at a public meeting and it was continued. Several small towns across the state engaged in "shotgun" quarantine; those who were unfamiliar to the men who stood at the quarantine station were asked to move on through the sight of a shot gun. This along with the lack of legal authority on the part of the Little Rock Board are two factors that would result in a call for a State Board of Health.

The hardest-hit towns were Helena, Hopefield (West Memphis) and Augusta on the White River. In Hopefield, there were 108 cases with 26 deaths.

There was a widely accepted idea in the 19th century that actions related to health and disease were local problems and it was only when it became apparent that local application of regulation was inadequate were they to be considered a state or national concerns. The Yellow Fever epidemic of 1878-1879 was an excellent case in point. Broad quarantines that affected the Caribbean Coast and the Mississippi River Valley were well beyond the resources of individual states and towns. In late 1878, the National Quarantine Act empowered the Surgeon General of the Marine Hospital Service to establish port quarantine on United States waterways. In 1879, the Congress created the first National Board of Health. It would last until 1883 when its funding was terminated. Despite its demise this marked a turning point in the need for public health action on a state and national basis.

The newly formed Arkansas Medical Society attempted to get the legislature to create a State Board of Health in the 1879 legislative session but was unsuccessful. Not to be deterred, the Medical Society created an unofficial State Board of Health as an arm of their organization and requested that the governor recognize them. This request languished on the governor's desk until another yellow fever outbreak in Memphis in the summer of 1879. He eventually accepted the request, pledging the state's "moral" support but no money. There were several reasons for this hesitation. First, and most important, the United States and Arkansas were in the middle of the Long Depression and the state was broke. Cotton prices had dropped from 50 cents a pound to 10 cents a pound and the tax coffers were empty. Secondly, the Medical Society represented the university-trained doctors and they were still looked at with a scrutinizing eye. Lastly, the doctors couldn't and didn't agree as to whether yellow fever was a contagious disease or not; this question would not be solved until the beginning of the next century.

Luckily for the people of Arkansas, the National Board of Health had been funded. After the governor's recognition, the now official State Board of Health applied for funds and received $7,500 in aid to deal with the new yellow fever threat.

Along with Memphis, Forrest City and Marianna dealt with significant outbreaks of yellow fever during the summer of 1879. The State Board set up quarantine stations along the Mississippi River and representatives of the State Board were dispatched to Forrest City, Hopefield and Marianna. As in other situations citizens who could, voted with their feet and left the towns. Eventually there was a cold spell and yellow fever faded into the background.

In 1881, the legislature jumped on the bandwagon and established an official State Board of Health. The legislation mandated the monitoring of disease, sanitary conditions and the accumulation of vital statistics. Despite this impressive mandate they provided only $3,000 a year for two years. Much like the National Board of Health, the Arkansas State Board of Health had no further funding after that first two years. As in earlier times it was viewed as a temporary necessity and only revived in times of crisis.

Cholera and yellow fever were the two diseases in the 19th century that created abject fear in the hearts of most Arkansans; both diseases came on rapidly and resulted in a violent, painful death in a short period of time. Smallpox caused a dreadful deforming illness but at least there was a vaccination that could be used. Infant death, malaria or ague, tuberculosis, scarlet fever, croup, eye diseases, whooping cough, measles, the flu, convulsions, typhoid, dysentery, worms, malnutrition and meningitis were all commonly reported. In the adult populations, gonorrhea and syphilis were a frequent complaint. To a great extent most of these illnesses were accepted as a part of daily life; illnesses for which little could be done. The periodicals of that time are full of advertisements for patent medicines and cures for the grip (flu), catarrh (chronic productive cough), rheumatism and lumbago, constipation, impotence, vermiague (worms) and tonics for energy. Despite the fact that significant advances were being made in identifying the basis of many of the infectious diseases that plagued people there was still little that could be done.

WOMEN, NURSING AND PROFESSIONALISM

By the 1880s, women had begun to have an impact on public life in Arkansas.

Until the 19th century female nurses were primarily nuns of religious orders. In the 1850s, pauper women in London were trained to go into the community and treat the poor becoming the first non-religious public health nurses. Florence Nightingale brought international attention to women as nurses beyond the home. Clara Barton helped to establish the American Red Cross which would have a large impact on crisis care in Arkansas during the twentieth century. A number of female lawyers and doctors began to have a presence in the state of Arkansas, such as Dr. A. T. Holton, the first woman doctor to open an office specializing in obstetrics in Little Rock in 1871. A budding Arkansas women's movement made itself known in the second half of the 19th century. Suffrage and the Women's Christian Temperance Movement played a prominent role. The State Teachers Association (all white) and the Colored Teachers Association were both formed by women in this timeframe. Women's Literary Guilds and Unions went well beyond their stated goals as women's clubs. The Ladies Benevolent Society of Little Rock funded and ran a charity hospital in Little Rock during the 1870s and 1880s. The Arkansas Chapter of the American Federation of Women's Clubs was formed in 1897 and played a powerful lobbying voice for the formation of the Arkansas Board of Health in 1913. In the early 1890s, Lillian Wald started teaching a home class on nursing for poor families in New York City. She was the first to use the term public health nurse to describe nurses whose work is integrated into the public community. Armed with statistics that demonstrated the value of nursing in illness, she convinced the Metropolitan Life Insurance Company to pay for her services. In 1916, Winifred Mann was one of the Metropolitan nurses working in the Fort Smith area as a visiting nurse.

Formal nurse training in Arkansas began at St. John's Hospital (now Sparks) in Fort Smith. The first class of three female nurses graduated in 1898. In 1901 the first nursing school in Little Rock was started at Logan H. Roots Hospital at the urging of the University of Arkansas Medical School. The matron of the school was Vinnie Middleton, an 1899 graduate of St. John's School. Eventually, Ms. Middleton became the wife of Dr. Charles Willis Garrison, the director of the Arkansas Board of Health. By 1914 there were four nursing schools in Little Rock; most of these nurses found work doing private duty in homes or accompanied individuals when they went to the hospital. In November 1912

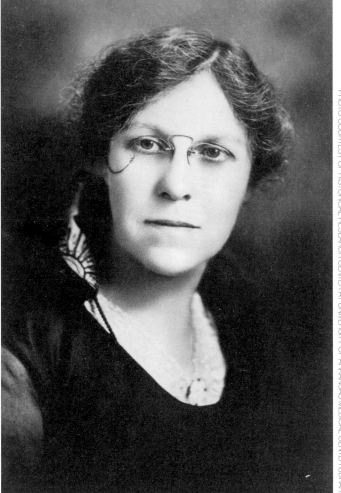

VINNIE MIDDLETON GARRISON WAS A GRADUATE OF ST. JOHN'S NURSING SCHOOL IN LITTLE ROCK. SHE WAS ACTIVE IN THE ARKANASAS FEDERATION OF WOMEN'S CLUBS AND WAS THE WIFE OF DR. CHARLES GARRISON WHO WOULD LEAD THE ARKANSAS BOARD OF HEALTH THROUGH ITS FIRST 20 YEARS.

FLORENCE NIGHTINGALE IS CREDITED WITH THE MODERN CONCEPT OF NURSING BEYOND THE CONFINES OF THE RELIGIOUS ORDER OR THE HOME.

IDA JO BROOKS WAS A POWERFUL, HEAD-STRONG FEMALE PHYSICIAN AND EDUCATOR WHO WAS A MAJOR PRESENCE IN ARKANSAS EDUCATION AND MEDICINE FOR 50 YEARS.

the Arkansas Graduate Nurse Association was formed and in 1913 a bill was passed in the legislature that required registration of nurses practicing in Arkansas and created a Board of Nurse Examiners. There were now two different levels of nurses: registered nurses and practical nurses. At this point in history the majority of the registered nurses were white and the majority of the practical nurses were black.

In 1912, Lillian Wald formed the National Organization for Public Health Nurses. Mary Breckinridge, one of the politically active members of the Arkansas Graduate Nurse Association, was an early member and was an outspoken proponent of public health nursing. Vinnie Middleton, Mary Breckinridge and Linnie Beauchamp were prominent voices in early nursing and in public health in Arkansas.

Present at the initiation of the nurse's organization was Dr. Ida Jo Brooks, a powerful, head-strong lady who had a major presence in Arkansas education and medicine for 50 years. Her father was Joseph Brooks of the infamous Brooks-Baxter war for Governorship of Arkansas in 1872. She obtained a bachelor's degree from Little Rock University, a master's from Drury in St. Louis in mathematics and by age 24 was the president of the Arkansas Teachers Association. In 1887, she applied to the University of Arkansas Medical School and was turned down because she was a female; not to be deterred she entered Boston University Medical School and in 1890 returned to Little Rock to practice pediatrics. In 1903, she returned to Massachusetts where she was trained as a psychiatrist and upon returning to Arkansas joined the staff of the State Hospital dealing in women's issues. In 1907, she became an assistant medical inspector for the Little Rock School district. She was instrumental in setting up medical evaluations of children in a school setting and in establishing the first classes in a school system in an Arkansas school for developmentally disabled children. In 1914 she became the first female physician to serve on the staff of the University of Arkansas Medical School.

The health care of the African-American population of Arkansas in the 19th century was a combination of self-help, some care provided by the white doctors of the state and black midwives. The problem with the care provided by the white physicians is that they suffered from a "moral astigmatism." They looked upon the blacks as a distinctively different and an inferior category of human beings. There were several diseases that were said to be only suffered by the black population, among them were: Cachexia Africana (dirt eating, now known to be associated with iron deficiency anemia), Struma Africana (tuberculosis) and Drapetomania (the disease which caused the slaves to run away). In the last half of the 19th century there were seven medical schools for the training of black physicians in the United States. The two that survived were Howard Medical School in Washington, D.C. and Meharry Medical School in Nashville; both schools also had dental schools associated with them. Most of the black physicians and dentists of Arkansas were trained at Meharry. The first documented black physician in Arkansas was Dr. Patience Brooks Trotter of Monticello. She was an herbalist who raised her own herbs and was highly valued by the black population and the white physicians alike. She specialized in those who suffered from cancer or "female problems." There were black physicians all around the state but most were in east Arkansas, where there was a large black population. Newport in Jackson County had a large number of physicians and dentists but the most successful black professionals centered on Helena. The black physicians and dentists were excluded by both the National and State Medical Societies so in 1893 they formed the Arkansas Medical, Dental, and Pharmaceutical Association.

In last half of the 19th century the towns and cities of Arkansas grew considerably. At the same time they became increasingly aware that behind many of the diseases they faced were invisible microorganisms that could be isolated. It became clear that the "taste test" for water quality was inadequate; the assumption had always been that if the water looked clean, didn't smell and tasted fresh, it must be fine. As early as the 1880s, public health labs began to spring up in the larger cities of the East. With the identification of bacteria as sources of disease, many of these labs shifted their focus from food purity to the culturing of bacteria. Practicing physicians continued to be skeptical about the idea of a germ for everything but by the early 20th century many of their objections had been overcome. It wouldn't be until the advent of the Arkansas Board of Health in 1913 that Arkansas would get its first bacteriologic lab.

During the last two decades of the 19th century, sanitation, water and sewage issues increasingly became topics of public debate. Without refrigeration, spoiled adulterated foods were a common problem. The city fathers of Little Rock had begun dealing with this issue in the 1830s. In 1879, Dr. C. E Nash, president of the State Board of Health listed adulterated foods as one of the major concerns. Filth in the streets, hog wallows in the center of town, dead animals, foul smelling bodies of water and small creeks that became open sewers are referenced repeatedly in the newspapers of the time. Springs that were adequate during the rainy season often dried up in the summer creating a need for more reliable water sources. For those who lived on a stream or river the answer was to dump their sewage into the stream. Little Rock would not stop dumping raw sewage into the Arkansas River until the 1960s. As a constituency for clean smelling air, safe water and disposal of waste grew, all of the towns across the state were eventually forced to deal with the issues.

Despite two long Depressions in the 1870s and the 1890s, a number of other positive changes were occurring. In the early 1870s, the Arkansas Medical Society began the process of forming a state wide organization. The Arkansas Dental Association formed in 1887. In 1887, Sparks Hospital was founded in Fort Smith. The following year, the Sisters of Charity opened Charity Hospital, now St. Vincent's Infirmary, in Little Rock. In 1859, the School for the Blind was founded in Arkadelphia and moved to Little Rock in 1968. The School for the Deaf was established in 1867. The Arkansas State Lunatic Asylum was opened and the first patients were admitted in March 1883. Two medical schools were established in Little Rock; one was a proprietary school started by a group of physicians and surgeons and the second was associated with the Arkansas Industrial University. A number of laws were passed regulating the practice of medicine, pharmacy and dentistry.

The same labs that discovered the various bacteria associated with the common epidemic diseases were continuing in their quest and turning their eyes toward producing vaccines and antitoxins to prevent these diseases. By the beginning of the 20th century, there were vaccines and antitoxins for smallpox, rabies, plague, cholera, and typhoid. However, no regulation of vaccine production existed. In 1902, the U.S. Congress passed the Biologics Control Act. This was the first major act designed to control the quality of drugs; it was enacted as a response to 1901 contamination events in St. Louis, Missouri and Camden, New Jersey involving smallpox vaccine and diphtheria antitoxin. In 1906, the Congress passed the Pure Food and Drug Act aimed at unlabeled and unsafe ingredients and misleading advertising.

The 19th century had been full of dramatic changes. The State of Arkansas had come a long way but there were still a number of unsolved problems. In 1901, after three quarters of a century of fighting between the "regular" physicians and the various eclectic groups of doctors, separate licensing boards were created for each discipline. In 1909, the requirement of a diploma for medical physicians ended the apprenticeship system. The two measures above created a pause in the battle between the various factions; but, soon they were at it again.

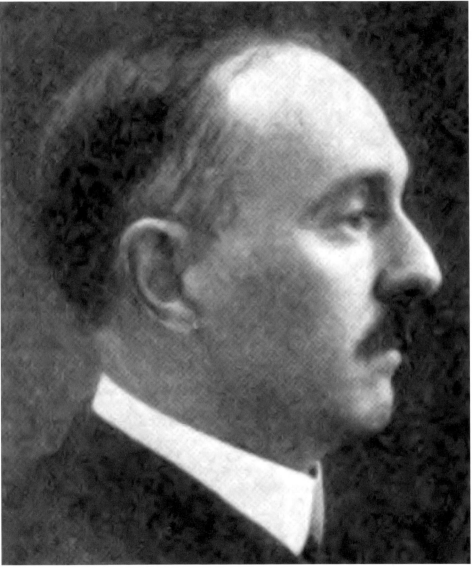

C-E.A. WINSLOW

CHAPTER FIVE
TIME TO PROGRESS

"Public health is the science and art of disease prevention, prolonging life, and promoting health and well-being through organized community effort for the sanitation of the environment, the control of communicable infections, the organization of medical nursing services for the early diagnosis and prevention of disease, the education of the individual in personal health and the development of the social machinery to assure everyone a standard of living adequate for the maintenance or improvement of health."

C-E.A. Winslow

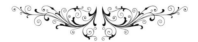

From the end of Reconstruction in 1877 until the beginning of the 20th century is considered the Gilded Age, a time of big business and trusts. The early 20th century saw the Progressive Era that focused on reform aimed at cleaning up politics, re-focusing the government, reining in the large trusts and improving the lot of the common man. Nationally, the rights of women and children became a major focus starting in the first decade of the new century. Sadly, Arkansas did not benefit from the Gilded Age except for the building of a railroad systems; it did, however, make progress during the Progressive Era. The health and welfare of the average citizen was one area that benefited.

The Arkansas economy that had languished during the last two decades of the 19th century began to wake up in the new century. Cotton, wheat and corn prices were on the rise. Crop diversification was occurring with increased production in rice and fruit such as apples and peaches and berries. Oil production in south Arkansas went through a boom starting in the second decade of the new century. Bauxite, coal and natural gas were being mined in various parts of west and central Arkansas. Timber production was up. A small but growing manufacturing sector was

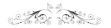

Judge Joseph Hill
of Little Rock:
"I have seen our
people dying among
strangers in a strange
land. I have seen
useless waste of
life, and I have seen
consumptives, under
proper care, return
to their families and
to lives of usefulness.
I know that the
establishment of
a sanatorium will
do more good
than any measure
pending before your
honorable body."

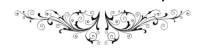

developing. This largess was not evenly distributed across the state: there were clearly class differences, racial differences and a significant gulf between those who lived in the cities (12.9 percent in 1910) and those who lived in a rural setting.

Child labor laws and child welfare made several steps forward in the first five years of the century but it was not until 1908 and the election of Governor George Donaghey that real progress began to be made. The people of Arkansas began to accept a wider definition of the services that the state could and should provide.

TUBERCULOSIS

During the first decade of the new century the first illness that came to the attention of those wishing to improve the health of Arkansas was tuberculosis. The disease is an ancient disease present in human population since the dawn of the Agricultural Age. As to when it became prevalent in the American South and specifically in Arkansas, no one knows for sure, but like malaria it probably emerged in the 17th century.

Consumption (tuberculosis) had been recognized as a common major illness since the early territory days of Arkansas. Prior to the 1880s and Dr. Robert Koch's discovery of the tuberculosis bacteria, it was assumed that TB was either a constitutional weakness on the part of the individual or was simply an untreated common lung problem gone awry. By the turn of the century almost everyone agreed that tuberculosis was an infectious disease and there was a strong association with poverty and malnutrition. In Western Civilization, the industrial revolution had concentrated large parts of the population in cities with inadequate housing and poor sanitation; this was associated with a dramatic increase in tuberculosis. Generally the first sign of significant disease was the coughing up of blood, followed by recurring fever and chills and then wasting (consumption). Even with the connection made between the bacteria and the illness, there was very little that could be done. Since there was no effective treatment the reasoning was that a regimen of rest and good nutrition offered the best hope for these patients. In 1863, the first tuberculosis sanatorium was opened in Poland. TB sanatoria became common throughout Europe from the late 19th century onward. In 1885 the Adirondack Cottage Sanatorium in New York State was the first such establishment in North America. In Switzerland, physicians believed that clean, cold mountain air was the best treatment for lung diseases so most sanatoria were built in isolated mountainous areas with clean fresh air away from the smog and grim of the cities.

In the early 20th century, tuberculosis sanatoria became common in the United States. In the early 1900s, Arizona's sunshine and dry desert air drew many people suffering from tuberculosis, rheumatism, asthma and various other diseases. For the rich there were TB resorts where people could go to take the cure. For those with no resources, TB camps in the desert were formed by pitching tents and building cabins.

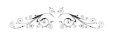

In 1912, Dr. Morgan
Smith, the father of
modern public health
in Arkansas described
the problem of
tuberculosis: "this
colossal ghost of
civilization is a social
question, and to be
solved it must be
prevented."

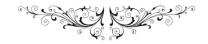

In 1905, Little Rock Judge Joseph Hill began to cough up blood and was soon diagnosed with active tuberculosis. He immediately moved to a sanatorium in Arizona where his disease was arrested and he was able to move back to Arkansas. He wrote a letter to the Arkansas House of Representatives: "I have seen our people dying among strangers in a strange land. I have seen useless waste of life, and I have seen consumptives, under proper care, return to their families and to lives of usefulness. I know that the establishment of a sanatorium will do more good than any measure pending before your honorable body."

In June 1908, Dr. A. T. Sweatland of the Arkansas Medical Society proposed that the state build a sanatorium and that the medical society form the Arkansas Tuberculosis Association. In January 1909, this organization was formed. The idea of a Christmas seal campaign had begun in Delaware in 1907. In 1908 the Arkansas chapter of the American Federation Women's Clubs picked up the idea and ran with it. The first public health nurses in Arkansas were TB nurses who were paid using Christmas seal funds. Like public health nurses after them they focused on examining children, diagnosing TB and educating the public about the dangers and prevention of this dreadful disease. In 1912, Dr. Morgan Smith, the father of modern public health in Arkansas described the problem of tuberculosis: "this colossal ghost of civilization is a social question, and to be solved it must be prevented."

Judge Hill was very persuasive man and in short order he became friends with State Senator Kie Oldham of Pulaski County who in 1909 authored the bill to create and fund the Arkansas Tuberculosis Sanatorium. Senator Oldham also had TB and would die of it in 1911. Tax funds were limited but they began work on the facility on a mountain top just south of Booneville and on August 10, 1910 the first patient was received. For 62 years, the Booneville facility grew and had a substantial impact on the people of Arkansas who had tuberculosis.

The bed space at the Sanatorium was doled out on a county by county basis and in the first four decades there was always a waiting list. The patients were divided up into those who were minimally ill, those with moderately advanced disease and those with advanced disease. Those with advanced disease had very little chance of surviving and most of the care was palliative. Those who came in at earlier stages of their disease often responded to enforced rest, good food and a quiet, calm atmosphere. At times as many as 85 percent of those with minimal disease left the sanatorium with a diagnosis of Arrested TB.

Another important impact of the sanatorium was the isolation of the sickest patients from the general population of the state.

Despite the fact that tuberculosis was common among the African-American population, there were no TB sanatorium beds for African-Americans in Arkansas until 1930 when the McRae Center in Alexander was

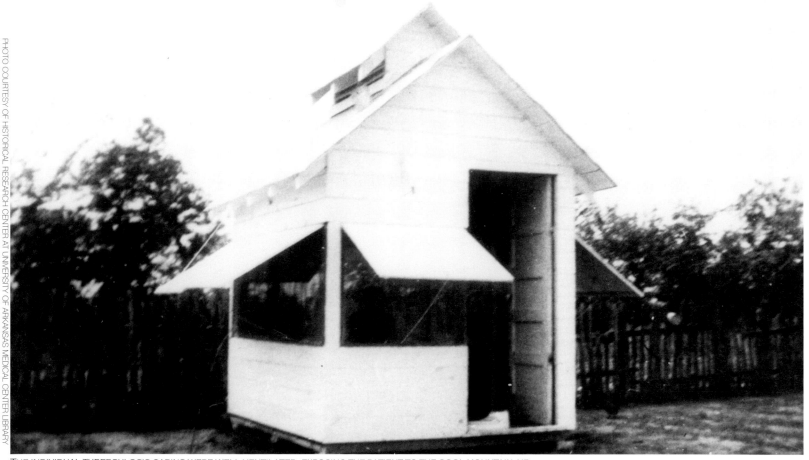

THE INDIVIDUAL TUBERCULOSIS CABINS WERE WELL VENTILATED, EXPOSING THE PATIENT TO THE COOL MOUNTAIN AIR.

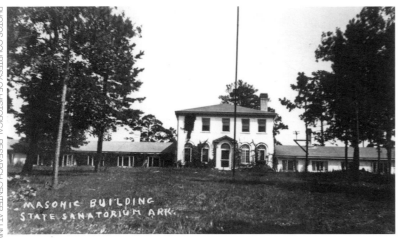

MASONIC BUILDING STATE SANATORIUM ARK.

THE MASONIC BUILDING WAS BUILT IN THE MID-1920S TO HOUSE AN INCEASING NUMBER OF CHILDREN WITH TUBERCULOSIS WHO PRESENTED TO THE SANATORIUM FOR CARE.

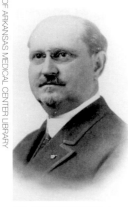

DR. MORGAN SMITH, A LEADER IN ARKANSAS MEDICINE FOR THE FIRST 30 YEARS OF THE 20TH CENTURY, WAS THE DRIVING FORCE BEHIND THE CONSOLIDATION OF TWO EXISTING MEDICAL SCHOOLS TO CREATE THE UNIVERSITY OF ARKANSAS MEDICAL SCHOOL AND WAS A LEADER IN THE DEVELOPMENT OF THE PERMANENT ARKANSAS BOARD OF HEALTH.

opened. Initially there were only 25 beds and for the duration of its existence it was always underfunded and the care was dismal.

Even with the racial component there was a growing constituency for improving the health of Arkansas that included an increasingly professionalism, better trained medical and nursing community, a more progressive political structure and an organization of politically active and interested women's groups.

The medical community of Arkansas was about to be dragged into the 20th century kicking and screaming. There is a degree of irony that the Progressive Era was in part a reaction to the large trusts and the "Robber Barons" of the late 19th century and it was two of those Titians of Industry who played a role in that process.

Andrew Carnegie and the Carnegie Foundation were commissioned by the American Medical Association to evaluate the state of medical education in the United States. Abraham Flexner was given the task of going around the country and doing surveys of all of the medical schools. Little Rock had two schools; one a proprietary institute owned by a number of doctors and the other was a small school loosely associated with the University of Arkansas.

Flexner's report stated that Arkansas had three times as many doctors as it needed and that neither of the medical schools had a single redeeming quality. After a series of bitter negotiations and a contentious legislative session, the University of Arkansas agreed to assume control of the combined schools. In 1911, the state legislature assumed fiscal responsibility and administrative control of the school. The next year, new quarters for the consolidated school were established in the Old State House with Dr. Morgan Smith as Dean.

THE GERM OF LAZINESS AND THE BOARD OF HEALTH

In 1902, Charles W. Stiles, a zoologist, reported that he had discovered "the germ of laziness," describing his studies of hookworm disease. At first he wasn't believed, the Dean of American medicine, Dr. William Osler of John's Hopkins, scoffed at the idea that hookworm was a major problem. Dr. Stiles was persistent and within a couple of years the medical profession was coming around. In 1909, Wicliffe Rose, director of John D. Rockefeller's charitable trust, convinced Rockefeller to provide $1 million for the formation of the Sanitary Commission for Eradication of Hookworm Disease. Under the direction of Rose, the commission undertook widespread testing, treatment, and education programs in 11 southern states.

To understand why it was called the "germ of laziness" we need to review the life cycle of the worm. Hookworm was a common infestation across the southern U.S. In the life cycle of the worm, the eggs are passed in human feces. The eggs mature into a larval form and then attach and penetrate the skin most often through bare feet. The larva then enters the blood stream and comes to a new resting place in the lung. This causes a form of "dry" pneumonia with a persistent cough. The worm then is expectorated and swallowed, finally implanting in the bowel wall of the human. Those who have a particularly heavy infestation often have severe forms of bleeding, weight loss, swollen feet, anemia, malnutrition and lethargy. Mental and physical development problems were common in growing children.

On initial surveys in the state it was apparent that one in five people in the state had hookworm in their stools. There is one reference stating that, in Hot Spring and Grant County, four of five people had the ubiquitous worm. The treatment was simple and harkens back to the days of heroic medicine. First the person was given something to purge them and then a dose of thymol to kill the worms. The patient was then given a second dose

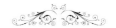

In 1902, Charles W. Stiles, a zoologist, reported that he had discovered "the germ of laziness," describing his studies of the hookworm disease.

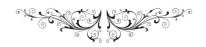

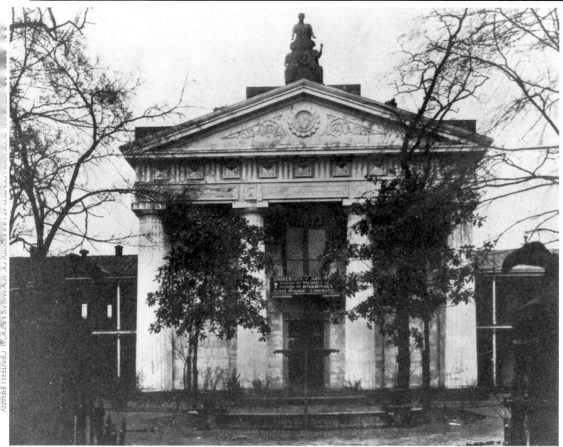

STATE GOVERNMENT HAD RECENTLY MOVED TO THE NEW CAPITOL. THE NEW CONSOLIDATED MEDICAL SCHOOL AND THE NEWLY FORMED STATE BOARD OF HEALTH SHARED THE OLD STATE HOUSE UNTIL THE MID-1920S.

of purgative to get rid of the mass of worm and the poison. Some cases were resistant and required more than one treatment cycle.

The prevention was even simpler: wear shoes and have a contained privy. A survey in 1912 of 7,500 homes in rural districts of the state showed that only 47 percent had ordinary outdoor toilets; 53 percent had no facilities at all.

There were several problems that had to be overcome.

The physician communities in the state were often not helpful and sometimes were openly resistant to outside help or anything that suggested change. In terms of immunization, hookworm control and later malaria and typhoid the best the authorities could hope for was that the physician population would not overtly fight them on these issues. A common refrain on the part of the medical community was that the prevention of the disease reduced the patient load of the physician. In 1910 Dr. Morgan Smith invited Dr. Stiles to come and address the state meeting of the Medical Society. Despite a good reception Smith and Stiles knew that those in attendance represented only a small number of the physicians in the state. Dr. Smith is quoted as having said: "You would be surprised to know how few of our

physicians know anything at all about hookworm disease. I have thought it getting the horse before the cart to educate the people in advance of the doctors and aim very careful not to antagonize the rural physicians." With that in mind, he organized a series of meetings around the state centered on the local medical societies.

The practical work of the hookworm commission was one of education, evaluation and treatment. Field physicians hired by the Board of Health conducted "dispensary campaigns" that resembled tent revivals. Flyers were sent out and advertisements bought in the local newspapers. Citizens were encouraged to bring a sample of their stool in a tin box labeled with their name and age. They would be treated on the spot and encouraged to come back to have their stool rechecked at a follow-up meeting. Brochures were provided strongly suggesting that children and adults wear shoes. Brochures and discussions of "scientific privies" were part of the overall package. Most of the brochures were heavy on pictures and simple diagrams.

The Rockefeller Foundation was hesitant to put money into a state that did not have a funded State Board of Health with a lab and an established Bureau of Vital Statistics. Since the State Board of Health was an on again/off again affair that had never been funded this provided a real difficulty for Smith. In 1911, he began a legislative campaign to create a funded State Board of Health and provide enough funds to match those of the Rockefeller Foundation. The biggest opposition came from a group known as the National League for Medical Freedom. This group included Eclectics,

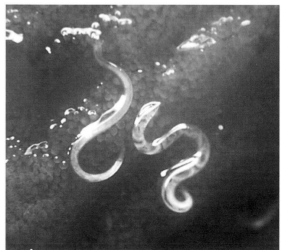

OVERALL, ONE IN FIVE ARKANSANS HAD HOOKWORMS. BUT IN SOME AREAS LIKE HOT SPRING AND GRANT COUNTY, FOUR OUT OF FIVE WERE INFECTED.

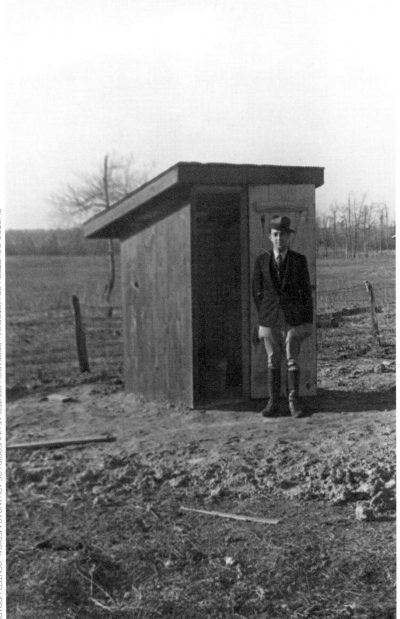

THE SOLUTION TO HOOKWORM WAS A WELL-CONSTRUCTED PRIVY AND WEARING SHOES.

this bill wanting to force all children to wear leather shoes. The legislation did pass both houses with the lobbying help of the Arkansas Federation of Women's Clubs and the encouragement of Governor Donaghey. Despite its passage, a series of nefarious maneuvers including the bill being lost before the governor could sign it and an alteration to the bill that the governor did sign resulted in the bill not becoming law. It would be two years later in 1913 that the legislature passed an almost identical bill and Arkansas had an official funded State Board of Health.

Though the hookworm program in Arkansas was only partially funded for the next two years with only the Rockefeller Funds and some modest county funds, the program generated a great deal of attention and provided valuable training for a young doctor who would lead public health efforts in Arkansas for the next 20 years.

Dr. Charles Willis Garrison was born in Bastrop County, Texas in 1878, attended Simmons College, Medical School in Galveston and then did an internship at the Memphis City Hospital; he practiced first in Tuscola, Texas and then Fort Smith, Arkansas. From his earliest time in medicine, he had a special interest in children's welfare and disease prevention. His wife, Vinnie Middleton Garrison, was a nurse who had been trained at St. John's Nursing School in Fort Smith in 1899 and by 1901 was the nurse matron at the Fort Logan Roots in North Little Rock. She was also active in the American Federation of Women's Club and very interested in child welfare. The Garrisons were both active in pushing for the establishment of a permanent State Board of Health. In 1911 Dr. Garrison was recruited by Dr. Morgan Smith, the State Sanitary Officer for Hookworm Eradication. Dr. Garrison became the Field Director for the Hookworm Eradication project and Dr. Smith's assistant. For the next two years he worked all around the state promoting, coordinating and dealing with the first statewide public health campaign. When the star-crossed Public Health Bill came up in the 1913 legislative session, Garrison was

helping to deal with a meningitis outbreak that began in the town of Lepanto and spread to other parts of the state. At that point Dr. Smith was still the executive secretary of the unfunded State Board of Health. Garrison acted as his eyes and ears in dealing with the epidemic.

The State Board of Health bill made it through the legislature a second time and went to the desk of Governor Joe T. Robinson; it sat there several days. There was a small epidemic of smallpox at which time the governor's office was bombarded by a letter writing campaign orchestrated by the

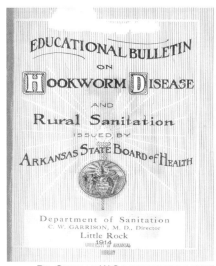

DR. CHARLES W. GARRISON WAS A TRUE BELIEVER IN EDUCATION WHETHER IT WAS TB, MALARIA, HOOKWORM OR VD.

Homeopaths, Christian Scientists and most important the patent medicine industry; it turned out that the patent medicine industry had a great deal of money they contributed to the fight. An interesting point that may have played a role was the fact that local newspapers across the country depended on patent medicine advertising as a major source of income. At one point a rumor was circulated that the leather industry from St. Louis was behind

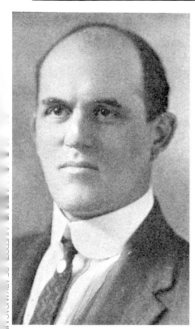

DR. CHARLES W. GARRISON, YOUNG PROTÉGÉ OF MORGAN SMITH, BECAME HEAD OF THE ARKANSAS BOARD OF HEALTH IN 1914 AND BUILT THE PROGRAM FROM SCRATCH.

Arkansas Federation of Woman's Clubs. He signed the legislation and Arkansas finally had a permanent, but poorly funded, State Board of Health.

Dr. Morgan served as the State Health Officer until May of 1914 followed by Dr. Frank Young who submitted his resignation after three months on the job. At this point the Rockefeller Foundation funding for the hookworm program was ceasing. Dr. Garrison was appointed as the new State Health Officer and Secretary of the Board of Health, positions he kept for 20 years.

Two other Progressive Era causes eventually dovetailed with the drive toward an overall approach to the health and welfare of the citizens of Arkansas: public education and a highway system for the state. In the first several decades of the 20th century, the county political and tax structure dominated these issues. The tax base for public health, schools and roads was based in the county and the taxes were based on assessed property values. The dominate political power lay with the large landowners and therefore property values were vastly under-assessed. This was especially true in the rural agricultural counties of south and east Arkansas and the remote mountain regions of the state. There was a strong feeling among the landowners and the powerful elite that educating workers, especially black workers, had almost no value and, in fact, was harmful. It was a major coup for education when in 1911 the Arkansas Educational Commission issued a statewide plan to strengthen education. Most of the plan was not implemented but there were perceptible improvements at least in white education in the first two decades of the 20th century. The road system of the state was a patchwork quilt of poorly built roads that were often impassible during the raining seasons of the year. Since money could only be expended in the district where it was collected, roads often ended at county or district lines. This lack of a system of roads added to the sense of isolation experienced by those who lived in the country and amplified the already existing distrust between those who lived in cities like Little Rock and Fort Smith and those in the country.

The public's health would be tied in many ways to education not only of the children of the state but the general populace and the physician community as well. Doctors Smith and Garrison clearly understood this issue and it would come to dominate an extended debate for most of the 20th century; prevention vs. curative, killing snakes vs. treating snakebites. It has been demonstrated repeatedly over the last two centuries that the practicing physician, treating one patient at a time with active disease, is not trained or inclined to promote population-based preventive health measures.

The broad categories of health problems that faced the average citizen had not changed dramatically in the last 70 years; the exceptions to this were the virtual disappearance of yellow fever and cholera. In the last years of the 19th century, yellow fever and malaria had become closely associated with mosquitoes. Cholera and typhoid were now clearly identified as water-borne diseases associated with poor sanitation; strategies for dealing with them, even when known, were seldom used. The TB sanatorium provided a ray of hope in dealing with the great white plague. An effective prevention for hookworm had been clearly demonstrated—wear shoes. Smallpox was common and vaccination was effective but there were major pockets of resistance among the population and the medical community against vaccination. Typhoid antitoxin was effective but not widely used. Epidemics of measles, meningitis, dysentery, typhoid, smallpox, whooping cough, scarlet fever, chickenpox, flu and diphtheria were common. Pellagra was common and, in the early part of the century, a debate still raged about whether it was an infectious disease or a nutritional deficiency disorder. Trachoma (chlamydia infectious of the eye) had been identified as an infectious disease and the blindness associated with it preventable. The use of a dilute solution of silver nitrate in the newborn's eye eliminated the disease; but, often it went unrecognized. Syphilis and gonorrhea were common and by World War I there was a non-mercury based treatment that was of marginal benefit at best.

The medical profession was beginning to make some progress especially in the area of surgery. The washing of hands, controlling for bleeding and gentleness with tissue were creating marked improvements in surgical mortality and morbidity numbers. In general, postpartum infections were disappearing in the white population. Most black women were still attended by black midwives, who though skillful in the delivery process, had not kept

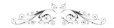

Dr. Smith is quoted as having said: "You would be surprised to know how few of our physicians know anything at all about hookworm disease. I have thought it getting the horse before the cart to educate the people in advance of the doctors and aim very careful not to antagonize the rural physicians."

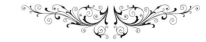

up in the area of hand washing and cleanliness; this, with the problem of malnutrition, resulted in a high incidence of infant mortality and puerperal infections. Orthopedics was still a mechanical job; the real advance was in open wounds and compound fractures. The idea of a clean wound and the prevention of infection had gone from a novel idea to a principle of care. The idea had not penetrated everywhere and for a good example, read T.E. Rhine, M.D.'s *Recollections of an Arkansas Country Doctor*. Dr. Rhine was a country doctor in Thornton, Arkansas. Several comments are made in the book about how Dr. Rhine always had a dirty rag in his back pocket that he used for all types of purposes. A Dr. Southhall in Fort Smith had begun experimenting with using irradiation of tissue for the treatment of skin problems. Dr. D. A. Rhinehart opened his office in the private practice of radiology in 1919 in Little Rock; he was the first to do X-ray and EKGs in his office.

There were a number of changes in equipment and medicines available to the physician during the first four decades of the 20th century. The paraphernalia used for bleeding, blister formation and cupping had been discarded by this time. The physician would have a ready supply of clean bandages and plaster material in the doctor's bag. There would be a modern stethoscope for listening to the chest. Depending on his level of sophistication he might have been a microcopist looking at urine, stool and sputum; though there was little he could do about the diseases themselves the microscope made him a better diagnostician. He had an array of surgical blades and steel instruments that at least gave the appearance of cleanliness. From a medicine standpoint he still had all of the standard chest rubs, nose drops, cough medicines and ointments that he compounded on the spot. Most of these had a strong odor or foul taste to add to their mystic. Continuing the heroic's love of heavy metals, calomel (mercury) was still used as a potent diuretic. Tincture of merthiolate (mercury) was introduced by Eli Lily in 1930 for painting wounds and scratches. It was unsuccessful until they added alcohol to make it sting and red vegetable dye to make it show on the skin. Syphilis was treated with Neosalvarsan, an arsenic based compound, that could be given intravenously.

Quinine was still the gold standard for malaria and its cousin quinidine for irregular heart rhythms, colchicine for gout, and nitroglycerin for heart pain. Digitalis for dropsy (heart failure) had come into common use. The doctor had benzocaine and procaine (local anesthetics), both second cousins to cocaine for anesthesia. He had opium and morphine for severe pain. Probably the most dramatic discovery and change in medicine was the development of injectable insulin for use in diabetics. From the time of its discovery in 1922 and mass production by E. J. Lilly Drug Company two years later, it became a mainstay in the physician's tool chest. The information float time was now down from decades to just two years. Sulfa drugs produced initially by Bayer Drug Company, made their emergence in the mid-1930s and almost immediately assumed widespread use.

BUILDING THE BOARD OF HEALTH

In 1914 when Dr. Garrison took over the Board of Health, the legislative act creating the board provided a broad poorly funded mandate. Under the leadership of Smith and Garrison, the new board established a comprehensive set of health rules and regulations based on identifying disease patterns and dealing with the root cause. They used as their model, rules created by several other states and the U.S. Public Health Services. Most important to the people of Arkansas was the development of a list of reportable infectious diseases and the creation of a Bureau of Vital Statistics to paint an accurate picture of the health and disease in the state and to begin looking at the quality of water and foods being offered to the public. As with education and public roads there was very little money to fund these services, but there were sources out there that could help and it was Garrison's job to find them.

Dr. Garrison's first challenge was smallpox. In 1915 smallpox was still a significant problem. Dr. Garrison remarked in a speech that there were 5,000 to 7,000 cases a year in the state despite the fact that there was an effective immunization available. In the summer of 1915, the county health doctor of White County, Dr. C. E. Holt, reported to the State Board that the town of Kensett had an ongoing outbreak of smallpox that had lasted for more than 12 months. With this information, the State Board issued an order that all employees, teachers and students show proof of immunization before they could report to work or attend school. This made Kensett the first school in Arkansas to require immunization for school attendance. Four months later, the town of Heber Springs became the second to require smallpox immunization. On December 3, 1917, based on a national recommendation from the U.S. Public Health Service, Arkansas was among the first states in the Union to introduce a compulsory vaccination program for all children starting school. In 1923, the first of two anti-vaccination challenges were launched. Both challenges were eventually struck down by the State Supreme Court. By the 1930s and 1940s, as a result of vaccination, smallpox had become an unusual occurrence.

Dr. Garrison's work with the Hookworm Eradication project created important contacts both up and down the chain of command. Working with the county judges and the various county medical societies gave him an understanding of the problems he faced and the areas where he would be welcomed. Going up the ladder he had developed personal contacts with the U. S. Public Health Service and the Rockefeller Foundation.

The next major project that faced Dr. Garrison and the new Board of Health was malaria. The disease had been endemic in Arkansas at least since the 17th century. Because of its prevalence it was generally accepted as a fact of life. It was not until the early 20th century that the association was made between mosquitoes and the disease.

In 1915, the Rockefeller Sanitary Commission for the Eradication of Hookworm morphed into the International Health Commission and turned its attention to malaria. During 1916, Garrison enticed the U.S. Public Health Service and the International Health Commission to create two demonstration projects in the state of Arkansas. Lake Village and Crossett were chosen to pursue two different approaches to the mosquito/malaria problem. Crossett, a company town, run by the Crossett Lumber Company welcomed the project with open arms. The town was plagued with mosquitoes and malaria. In 1916 a survey created a map showing all of the mosquito breeding sites. During the summer, workers cleaned the ditches and streams and oiled the bodies of standing water. The results were remarkable. In one year, the doctor's calls for malaria dropped 90 percent. The total cost of the project was $1.45 per person; less than the cost of a physician's office visit.

A different approach was taken in Lake Village; here the project centered on educational efforts, installing window screens in homes and treating identified human carriers with quinine. The results in Chicot County were equally as impressive. The numbers testing positive for malaria dropped by two thirds while the incidence of malaria remained the same in the rest of

the county. Similar to Crossett the cost came to a total of $1.80 per person.

In 1916, the St. Louis Southwestern Railroad began a series of projects of malaria control along their rail lines in Arkansas with equally gratifying results.

WORLD WAR I, THE U.S. PUBLIC HEALTH SERVICE AND THE FLU

In April 1917, the United States entered World War I and, by May, the government was looking for locations to establish cantonments for military troops. Camp Pike (presently Camp Robinson) was picked as an ideal location

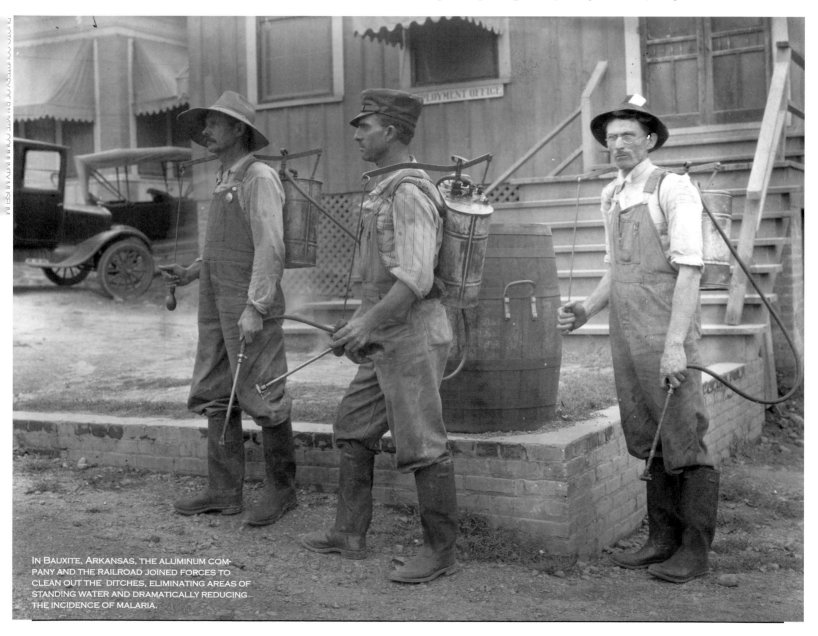

IN BAUXITE, ARKANSAS, THE ALUMINUM COMPANY AND THE RAILROAD JOINED FORCES TO CLEAN OUT THE DITCHES, ELIMINATING AREAS OF STANDING WATER AND DRAMATICALLY REDUCING THE INCIDENCE OF MALARIA.

in the center of the country. Ever aware of an opportunity to bring forces to bear on the health of Arkansas, Garrison worked closely with a group of generals and civic leaders in developing the site. The one objection to the site was the potential of malarial conditions. He convinced the Army along with the U.S. Public Health Service into putting a significant amount of money into the site and using the Camp and the extra-cantonment area (Pulaski County) as a demonstration area similar to what had been done in Crossett and Lake Village. Working with J.C. Geiger, Assistant Epidemiologist, R.E. Tarbett, Sanitary Engineer, and C.C. Pierce, Assistant Surgeon General, they developed a plan to improve the health of not only the troops at Camp Pike but the general citizenry of central Arkansas. This eventually extended to Lonoke County with the establishment of Eberts Field, an army training air field.

The areas of work included malaria control, general communicable disease, venereal diseases, school inspections, control over production and sale of milk, control over production of food and drink, control over barber shops and manicure shops, rural sanitation, general sanitation, public health nursing, laboratory services and education. It is quite interesting that this list of items coincides closely with the state mandate set up for the State Board of Health. The statistics accumulated and outcomes of this two year project informed the public health efforts for decades.

Malaria was the first problem to deal with. Using the results of the studies done in Crossett, Lake Village and other towns across the South they cleared the standing water, oiled the small bodies of water and within a year the incidence of malaria both in the cantonment area and the extra-cantonment area were reduced by 90 percent.

Except for minor outbreaks of measles, German measles, meningitis and the Flu Epidemic of 1918, the standard panel of communicable diseases was well controlled. They instituted an aggressive campaign of smallpox and typhoid immunization. Approximately 50,000 doses of smallpox vaccine and typhoid vaccination were given. At that time this was probably the largest population coverage in any one community, anywhere. In the first year of the project, there were 600 cases of smallpox reported and in the second year zero. There were two minor outbreaks of typhoid and each was related to food contamination. In each case, rapid epidemiologic investigation proved the source to be unpasteurized milk or ice cream.

Thirty-six percent of those young men in Arkansas taking induction physicals were found initially unfit for duty. Tuberculosis, malnutrition and venereal disease, specifically syphilis and gonorrhea, were among the most common problems. Ninety-plus percent of the venereal disease during the war was determined to have been preexisting before the service men came into the ranks. The incidence among the black soldiers was eight to 10 times as high as among the whites. This would be the first war where accurate diagnosis could be made and reasonably effective treatment administered. Many of the soldiers were offered treatment and then re-tested. The aggressive dealing with houses of prostitution and the development of an isolation ward at the University Medical School for those found to be carriers of disease were effective in reducing the rate of disease. An aggressive campaign designed to

teach and scare the troops was used as well.

Control over milk, food and drink products offered to the public were aimed at looking at the food and drink chain from the raw product to consumption. Major inroads were made in reducing the bacteria count in the milk and other food products. There were two primary milk sources for the military base; one was local and another in Prairie and Lonoke counties. Three hundred dairies were involved in the Prairie and Lonoke counties. Many of the cattle were poor milk producers and there were major problems with a partial pasteurization process to prevent spoiling. In the end, Camp Pike imported and raised its own cow herd to supplement what it was getting locally.

Prior to this study, the only medical inspection of the local schools was being performed by Dr. Ida Jo Brooks in the Little Rock school system. She was appointed an Acting Assistant Surgeon of the Public Health Service and assigned several nurses to help her expand her work to North Little Rock and the rural districts of the county. Over 6,000 children were examined and 3,500 defects were found. During the first year of the project, a dental clinic was set up in the school system. This represents the first significant evaluation of the health of school children in Arkansas.

At the beginning of this project, there was one Red Cross nurse and, by the end of the second year, there were eight nurses working. This occurred as the U.S. Public Health acted to coordinate the visiting nurses scattered around the county. Much of their work involved convalescent care and school medical exams; 38 percent of their work related to tubercular care.

The laboratories of the city of Little Rock, the Board of Health and the Medical School were inadequate to handle the work load presented by the project as it progressed. The U. S. Public Health service provided extra equipment and a temporary second bacteriologist. Eventually the Red Cross provided an appropriation and a replacement bacteriologist.

The last and certainly not the least important element of this study were the sanitary and rural sanitation work. They inspected homes, schools, restaurants, hotels, water supplies and sewer systems. One-fourth of the homes in Little Rock were using privies and not connected to a water system. In North Little Rock, one-half to two-thirds were using privies and not connected to a water system. Rural sanitation was aimed at the areas around Camp Pike and the protection of the water supply to the camp. Most of those activities focused on education and attempting to entice the residents to use properly constructed privies.

The results of the study and the work done in the Central Arkansas region demonstrated what could be done in a short period of time. Most of the services provided were inexpensive and simply required the political will and cooperation of all of those involved. In the end, the study clearly pointed out the many problems that faced the citizens of Arkansas; it also pointed the way for Dr. Garrison and his people.

World War I was reasonably short lived for the people of Arkansas. In this deadly war, the general causality count was high because of the type of fighting involved. Despite this, only 2,200 troops from Arkansas lost their lives in the fighting. From a historical perspective, this was the first war where more men were killed by enemy fire than by illness and disease. Because of advances in surgery, cleanliness and general sanitation, the odds were good that a solider would survive the post-battle recuperation.

The home front was not as lucky. In the fall of 1918, the state of Arkansas was hit by what came to be known as the Spanish Flu. The name Spanish Flu came from the fact that most warring countries did not report their civilian mortality statistics but Spain did since it was not a combatant. Flu had been a common illness in Arkansas since the territorial days but there was something different about this version. Speculation is that the virus went through an immunologic shift or drift resulting in the inability of the human population to demonstrate any immunity to the agent. It is felt that it probably originated in Kansas and spread around the world from there. Worldwide the 1918 flu killed more people in a year than the Bubonic Plague did in 100 years. More than 600,000 Americans and 7,000 Arkansans died. More Arkansans died in a short time from this epidemic than any other epidemic since the days of the European introduction of smallpox and measles to the American Indians. The two leaders of public health in Arkansas at the time were Dr. Garrison and J.C. Geiger, the U. S. Public Health epidemiologist at Camp Pike. Despite concerns, their first response was to reassure the population and advise masking, coughing into a handkerchief and avoiding crowds. Over a two week period the situation worsened and, in early October, Dr. Garrison and the Board of Health imposed a statewide quarantine closing schools, churches, theaters and lodges. Short of quarantine, there was very little that could be done. Most of the deaths occurred in young reasonably healthy people. The course was usually one of high fever, muscle aches and headache followed by the development of pneumonia. A significant number of those who developed pneumonia died. After the war ended on November 11, the quarantine was lifted. No part of the state was spared from the epidemic. For the next year, small outbreaks occurred around the state especially in the rural sections. The one interesting exception was the TB Sanatorium in Boonville, Arkansas. Early on the self-contained facility enforced a strict quarantine and there were no cases of flu among the patients or staff.

With smallpox, World War I and the flu behind them Dr. Garrison went about putting a team together to deal with the other pressing problems of health and disease of Arkansas.

By 1919, a number of the counties had part-time public health physicians. At this point, all of these men were practicing physicians in the community who were usually friends with the county judge. They provided care for the prisoners and did a certain amount of charity work for the poor. On occasion they were called on to intervene in a health problem related to school. Any compensation they received was minimal.

The first bureau to be established by the Board of Health was the Bureau of Vital Statistics. Initially headed by Nell Smart, she was replaced in 1916 by Mary Ellis Brown. The plan was to establish a registrar for all births, deaths and divorces in each county and this information was to be funneled to the state bureau. For several years there was confusion as to who was to pay for these services. It would be the 1930s before reliable data would begin to be accumulated. When the public health nurses began to make forays into the rural counties, they found that a large number of the births were either not recorded or not forwarded to the state bureau. During the Flood of 1927, the Red Cross had trouble making heads or tails of the data they were accumulating because of the lack of a good statistical base. The first death certificate recorded in the bureau was from Stuttgart in Arkansas County and the cause of death was malaria.

It appears that Garrison hoped to use the data developed during the war to push the political structure of the state to pursue several of the problems pointed out by the Camp Pike Project. One of the first extensions of the Camp Pike Project was legislation for the licensure and inspection of hotels, rooming houses and restaurants. A second issue was the extent of venereal disease in the United States and Arkansas. In 1919 federal appropriations were made to continue the work done in North Little Rock. A large VD clinic run by the U. S. Public Health Service was established in Hot Springs and continued to function for two decades under the leadership of Dr. Oliver Wenger.

One of the unsung heroes of this era was M. Zach Bair, the first Sanitary Engineer for the State of Arkansas. Mr. Bair arrived in 1919 in the wake of World War I and the Camp Pike project in North Little Rock. He was a quiet, soft spoken engineer who was averse to politics. A native of Pennsylvania, he was educated at John's Hopkins and Cornell, and worked as the Assistant Sanitary Engineer in the State of Ohio before coming to Arkansas. One of the first extensions of the Camp Pike Project was legislation for the licensure and inspection of hotels, rooming houses and restaurants. Bair's primary charge from the Arkansas Board was to evaluate the state of water and sewer systems in the state. An initial survey revealed that there were 58 municipal water supplies in the state supplemented with 70 railroad water supplies. There were only 35 sanitary sewage systems in the state. Almost all of the water and sewer systems were faulty and in his words, "a serious menace to the health of the community." He tended to be rather matter of fact in his comments. Early in his career there was a typhoid epidemic in Eureka Springs that seemed to center on the Basin Street Spring. There were

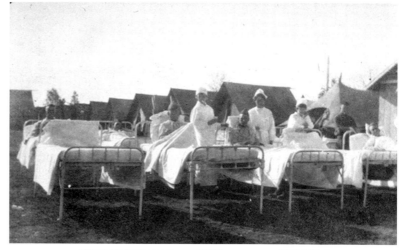

WITH THE SPANISH FLU IN 1918 MORE THAN 600,000 AMERICANS AND 7,000 ARKANSANS DIED.

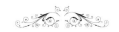

ZACH BAIR WAS THE FIRST SANITARY ENGINEER EMPLOYED BY THE STATE BOARD OF HEALTH.

a number of houses on the hill side above the spring none of which had a scientific privy. He discovered that the spring was quite polluted and was the probable source of the typhoid. The city fathers asked what could be done. His comment was unless the homes above the spring were eliminated they would need to dynamite the spring. He wasn't invited to return to Eureka Springs. The reason that most municipalities had no water or sewer source was the upfront cost of getting a system up and running. With the blessing of the Board of Health, Bair helped to draft legislation for the issuing authority for revenue bonds which made local water and sewer projects possible. During his 18-year tenure, the number of modern water systems in the state increased from 58 in 1919 to 173 in 1937. He and his staff were available to help cities develop the specifications for local systems. He helped the city of Little Rock develop their overall plan for water and sewer that resulted in the building of Lake Winona on the Alum Fork of the Saline River; this acted as sole clean water source for Central Arkansas starting in 1938 and remained as such until Lake Maumelle was completed in 1958. In 1937, he left the Board of Health and started a private engineering firm aimed at assisting communities in the state. In the 1940s, he developed active tuberculosis and died in 1947 at the Boonville Santorum.

PUBLIC HEALTH NURSING

Public Health Nursing developed over several decades. Starting in 1908 and the establishment of the Arkansas Tuberculosis Association, nurses began to transition from private duty and hospital nursing to a more active role in the community. One of the initial problems to be overcome was how these nurses would be paid. The first sources of revenue to finance this work came from the Christmas Seal campaign, Metropolitan Life Insurance and a number of charities the most important of which was the Red Cross. Pushed by Erie Chambers, the executive director of the TB Association, the Christmas Seal campaign was pursed by the Arkansas Federation of Women's Club and provided funds for nurses to go into the communities around the state examining and identifying those with TB. Metropolitan Life Insurance Company, using statistics accumulated by Lillian Wald of the National Visiting Nurse Association, demonstrated the economic value of in-home nursing during illness. In 1916, Winifred Mann of Fort Smith was one of several Metropolitan nurses working in the state. The Mississippi Flood of 1912-1913 marked the first presence of the American Red Cross in Arkansas. During World War I the Red Cross provided nursing services at Camp Pike and in the extra-cantonment area of Pulaski County. It would be 1917 before the first Red Cross Chapters formed in the state: the first was in Garland County and second in northeast Arkansas the following year.

In addition to the financing, each of these organizations added a number of pieces to the jigsaw puzzle that is public health nursing. The tuberculosis nurses provided a framework that functioned in the county-centered politics of the state. Entry to the TB sanatorium was parsed out on a county-by-county basis and required the cooperation of the county judge in addition to some financing. The insurance nursing data provided facts for the effectiveness of the work. The Red Cross Nursing services brought with them professionalism and a national team of support with influence in high places.

Linnie Beauchamp is one of the heroes of our story. She was born on April 23, 1891 in the small town of Wheatly, Arkansas just west of Forrest City. She was the daughter of Dr. Nicholas Prince Beauchamp, a country doctor who worked with Dr. Cummings of Forrest City during the yellow fever outbreak of 1879. She graduated from the Crowley's Ridge Institute with honors and went on to get her diploma in nursing from the City Hospital of Memphis. During her training she worked on the TB and typhoid wards. After her training she went to work with the TB association in Shelby County, Tennessee as the Executive Secretary in charge of the Christmas Seal campaign. During World War I she worked in extra-cantonment zones around military camps in Alabama and was active in the flu epidemic of 1918. After the War she received extra training from the Red Cross to qualify her as a nurse supervisor for Red Cross. In 1918, the head of the St. Louis Red Cross office brought her to Little Rock, introduced her to Dr. Charles Garrison of the Arkansas Board of Health and in her own words: "handed me to him on a silver platter, as they say, with my full salary, the full salary of a secretary—if I could find one suitable—and an office and equipment to set up a program of developing and promoting Red Cross county health nursing services under the direction of the State Health Department but financed by the Red Cross." And so public health nursing of Arkansas had begun.

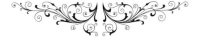

In 1919, almost all of the water and sewer systems in Arkansas were faulty and in Zach Bair's words: "a serious menace to the health of the community."

As soon as Ms. Beauchamp set up her office, she began recruiting from the nursing schools around the state. One of the requirements of the Red Cross was that anyone working under their umbrella had to have a three month program of public health nursing education. This slowed the process down to some extent. The first two counties to have nursing placements were Newport in Jackson County and Russellville in Pope County. An additional requirement was that each nurse must work under an active nursing committee; these committees were composed of representatives of private health agencies, women's clubs, the county judge, the department of education and the county medical society. By 1921, Pope, Jackson, Union, Ashley, Washington, Miller, Clark County Monroe, Hot Spring, Bradley, Craighead and Phillips Counties all had public health nursing.

While Dr. Garrison and Ms. Beauchamp were toiling away at developing an active public health nursing service in the state of Arkansas, there were movements afoot on a national basis that aided this process along. At the beginning of the 20th century, six to nine women out of every 1,000 live-births died from complications, 112 children out of 1,000 live-births died before the age of one year and most of these deaths were preventable; the numbers for black women and children were double that for whites. Perinatal infection, infant diarrhea, malnutrition and poverty were four of the big causes. Despite not having the right to vote, women's voices had begun to be heard. In 1912 during the heyday of the Progressive movement, a Federal Children's Bureau was formed as the primary agency aimed at improving the health of mothers and children. One of the first findings of this Bureau was that 80 percent of pregnant women received no advice or trained care. These numbers were worse in rural areas and there were major racial discrepancies. The Women's Movement in the United States resulted in the 19th Amendment (women's right to vote) to the Constitution in 1919 and its ratification in 1920. In 1921 the Sheppard-Towner Act (Promotion of Welfare and Hygiene of Maternity and Infancy Act) was passed and signed into law. States were allowed to opt in or out of the program but to be in the program they were required to establish a Children's Bureau and match the Federal Governments funds up to $5,000. The American Medical Society and the Arkansas Medical Society were dead set against this bill and fought against it. Despite its positive results they continued to lobby against the bill and by 1929 the funding for the act was allowed to lapse. There was however a split in the larger doctor's organization, the pediatric section of the American Medical Association came out in support of the Act in 1929 and this resulted in the creation of the American Academy of Pediatrics.

Linnie Beauchamp read *Good House Keeping* religiously. She noticed an article that described a traveling examination clinic sponsored by the Federal Children's Bureau and manned by Dr. Frances Sage Bradley. She took the article to Dr. Garrison who in turn called the Federal Bureau. After a series of calls, telegrams and letters, Dr. Bradley and her truck were in Arkansas. At the end of the legislative session in 1922 she spoke to a joint session and apparently impressed the group. The ordinarily tight-fisted legislature agreed to participate in the program, establish a Children's Bureau and match the federal funds. Dr. Bradley became the head of the Arkansas Children's Bureau and

began traveling the state with her medicine show. The road system in the state was extremely poor and limited creating major mechanical problems for her truck and making penetration into some parts of the state difficult. During her stay in the state she held nine child health conferences and invited the public. While in the state Dr. Bradley covered a total of 18 counties and began to make inroads into the maternal and infant care. She, Linnie Beauchamp and Agnes McCall did a survey of children's health in Bradley County and found large numbers of preventable health defects among the rich and poor children; chief on the list were malnutrition and dental problems. Two public health nurses were hired and charged with the task of investigating the practice of midwifery and the under-registration of births. Like Dr. Garrison, Bradley was convinced that education was the most important preventive tool that they had. She created nine pamphlets called the Arkansas Family Series. She and her nurses were not always welcomed with open arms. She related one story in a letter to her daughter about an encounter at one of her health meetings. "One old fellow (a doctor) glared at me when I insisted that a good public health nurse in each county would prove more helpful to the mothers than adding another doctor. This made him froth at the mouth but the rest of the crew kidded him when I reminded him that the mothers needed to be shown how to bake decent bread for their families, how to prepare milk in ways sufficiently attractive to break up the coffee habit they had taught their children; how to cook grits, soup and field peas, and (that) there are other ways of serving meat and vegetables than frying."

Though her tenure was short, Dr. Bradley's medical evangelism was contagious and set the tone for public health nursing for the next several decades. In November 1923, she resigned after a dispute with Dr. Garrison over publication of the pamphlets she had created and control over the

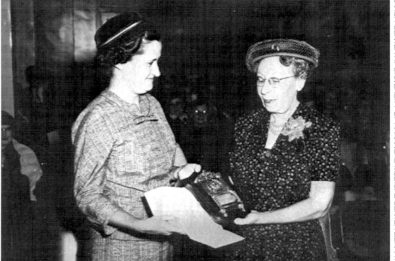

A QUOTE FROM LINNE BEAUCHAMP REGARDING HER INTRODUCTION TO DR. CHARLES GARRISON BY THE HEAD OF THE ST. LOUIS RED CROSS OFFICE: "HANDED ME TO HIM ON A SILVER PLATTER, AS THEY SAY, WITH MY FULL SALARY, THE FULL SALARY OF A SECRETARY — IF I COULD FIND ONE SUITABLE — AND AN OFFICE AND EQUIPMENT TO SET UP A PROGRAM OF DEVELOPING RED CROSS COUNTY HEALTH NURSING SERVICES UNDER THE DIRECTION OF THE STATE HEALTH DEPARTMENT BUT FINANCED BY THE RED CROSS." AND SO PUBLIC HEALTH NURSING OF ARKANSAS HAD BEGUN.

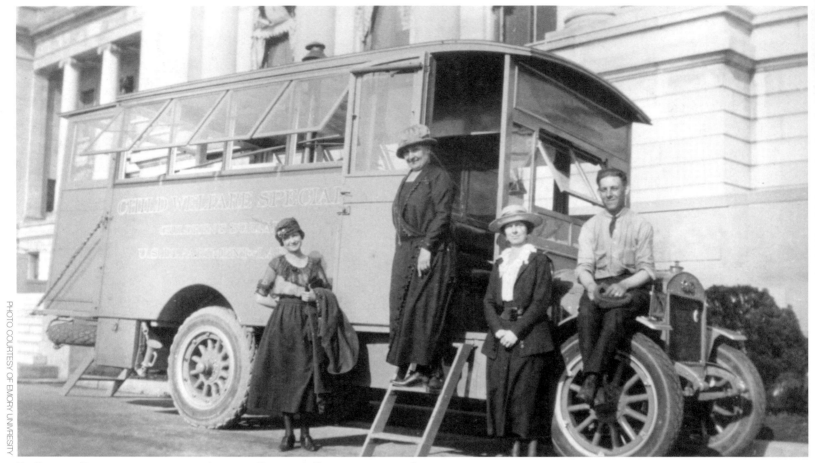

DR. FRANCES BRADLEY WAS HEAD OF THE ARKANSAS CHILDREN'S BUREAU FOR A YEAR. SHE AND HER CREW TOURED THE STATE FOR A YEAR DEALING PRIMARILY WITH INFANT AND MATERNAL ISSUES. SHE LEFT AFTER A CONFLICT WITH DR. GARRISON.

Children's Bureau.

Her departure did not change the course of the maternal and infant care approaches in Arkansas. The next several years saw a dramatic increase in the number of public health nurses in the state. By late 1924 there were 24 nurses actively engaged in public health activities and those numbers continued to grow.

The Arkansas Children's Home Society began as an orphanage in 1912. In 1916, retired Methodist minister Dr. Orlando P. Christian was named superintendent. Throughout the 1920s the orphanage slowly grew. Initially children in need of acute medical care were first treated by St. Vincent's until they were medically stable and then moved to the home. Despite the home teetering on the edge of financial disaster, a new children's hospital was opened in 1926. In 1934 Ms. Ruth Beall took over as superintendent of the facilities. Both Dr. Christian and Ms. Beall let it be known to the nurses on the front lines that they would help in any way they could.

Two significant problems uncovered by the public health nurses entering the schools and examining students were the number of children with physical defects and blindness.

The nurse narratives of Linnie Beauchamp, Ruby Kincaid and Mary Emma Smith are full of references to the numbers of children with spina bifida, paralysis secondary to polio and club feet. Ms. Beauchamp describes a number of late night trips along rough, country roads, taking young ill children to Little Rock and depositing them in the arms of Children's hospital.

Blindness was another issue. As early as 1918, Dr. W.T. McCurry of the School for the Blind presented a paper before the Medical Society stating that there were 110,000 people in the state of Arkansas who fit the legal definition of blindness and 25,000 of those cases were completely preventable. A large number of those cases were caused by ophthalmia neonatorium (gonorrhea infection of the eye at birth) and trachoma (chlamydia infection of the eye). The instillation of copper sulfate drops for the first and sliver nitrate drops for the second dramatically reduced the probability of blindness. Once either infection became embedded they were difficult to control.

Since a high percent of women, especially rural women, had no prenatal care or assistance with delivery, many children did not receive this simple remedy.

The clear identification of those women who were carriers of gonorrhea

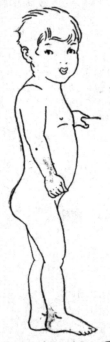

"It's great to be born in Arkansas"

THE ARKANSAS FAMILY SERIES

8. *Concerning the Baby*
STATE BOARD OF HEALTH
and
U. S. DEPARTMENT OF LABOR
CHILDREN'S BUREAU
COOPERATING

DR. BRADLEY WROTE A SERIES OF PAMPHLETS AIMED AT EDUCATION OF MOTHERS ABOUT THE CARE AND TREATMENT OF THEIR CHILDREN.

was difficult and would have represented the real primary prevention but that would not occur for another two decades.

Trachoma was thought to be primarily a problem of the mountain people of northwestern Arkansas. With the advent of sulfonamides in the 1930s, trachoma eventually disappeared from the United States, except for pockets of Native Americans and parts of the Appalachians. In the early 1920s, a Red Cross Public Health Nurse named Ms. Leonard, working in Ashley County near Hamburg, came upon a number of women who were blind as were their children. These women's eyes were chronically inflamed and watered profusely. Most had been treated by local physicians and told there was

nothing else that could be done. She was able to convince her superiors to pay to take one of these women to Memphis to see Dr. E. C. Ellet, an eye surgeon. When Dr. Ellet looked at the woman the first word out of his mouth was: "Trachoma." This woman and her children had trachoma. He operated on the woman and was able to partially restore her sight; more important he was able to render her non-infectious to others. When Dr. Garrison was informed of the diagnosis, he contacted Dr. Ellet and then the U. S. Public Health Service. A trachoma specialist was sent to Arkansas to do a survey of Ashley County in south Arkansas and the mountainous regions of north Arkansas. This survey confirmed the presence of significant pockets of trachoma in the state. There was already in existence a trachoma hospital in Rolla, Missouri; a branch of that hospital was opened in Russellville, Arkansas. The public health nurses of north Arkansas became attuned to signs of trachoma. During the early part of the Depression funding dried up and the Russellville hospital closed. By the late 1930s, sulfa drugs became available and in 1941, Dr. K. W. Cosgrove Sr., a graduate of the University of Toronto, Canada who was teaching eye, ear, nose and throat medicine at University of Arkansas in Little Rock, almost singlehandedly wiped out trachoma in Arkansas. In one year, he treated 2,611 cases with surgery, drops and oral sulfa saving 83 percent of those patients from sure blindness.

This is another instance where treatment became a point of contention between the private physician community and public health. The physicians of Ashley County complained bitterly to Dr. Garrison about the nurse stepping over the line and invading their territory regardless of the positive outcome.

THE FLOOD OF 1927

On Friday, April 15, 1927, the first break in the Arkansas Levee system occurred on the Arkansas River in western Arkansas. The next day a levee at Marked Tree on the St. Francis River collapsed. On Thursday, April 21, 1927, the levees along the Mississippi River broke and began inundating the Delta. The river levels along the Mississippi, Arkansas and White Rivers had been high for months. In one day, seven inches of rain fell in Little Rock. All of the streams and lakes were full and the land was saturated. When the levees broke, the rivers took back what they had owned for millennia. Thirty-six of the 75 counties in the state and most of the rich agricultural land were covered with water and those who lived there were forced to scramble for safety. In the end, 98 lives were lost in the acute flooding and 143,000 people were forced from their homes.

Most of the society of the Delta was composed of a few rich white landowners and a large number of white and black sharecroppers. Land value and cotton prices had dropped dramatically in 1920s. Synthetic fibers were making inroads in the clothing industry. Boll weevils and red spiders had almost destroyed several cotton crops. The economy of the farm was controlled by the men who owned the mercantiles, banks, sawmills and cotton gins; forms of peonage were commonplace and in some areas ruthlessly enforced. Education was discouraged because it was thought to interfere with a pliant workforce. Healthcare when available was often provided through the

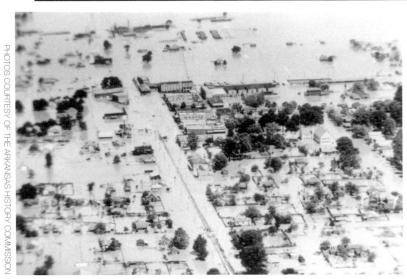

THIRTY-SIX OF THE 75 COUNTIES IN THE STATE AND MOST OF THE RICH AGRICULTUR-AL LAND WERE COVERED WITH WATER AND THOSE WHO LIVED THERE WERE FORCED TO SCRAMBLE FOR SAFETY.

landowner and then begrudgingly. Almost all deliveries were done by poorly trained midwives. For long periods of the year, the diet was composed of salt meat, corn meal and molasses. Malnutrition in several different disguises was common especially pellagra and scurvy. Most of the Delta counties had been slow to embrace any form of public health.

President Coolidge appointed Herbert Hoover, his Commerce Secretary and an expert in disaster relief, to oversee the relief work in the Mississippi Valley. His first response was to turn to the Red Cross and the Rockefeller Foundation. To accommodate the refugees, the Red Cross set up a total of 80 aid camps in Arkansas. The Forrest City Camp in St. Francis County had a record number of 15,850 displaced persons at its height. When they entered the camp, each person was required to receive an identification card to obtain clothing and food. All were given smallpox and typhoid immunization. Estimates are that more than 50,000 sets of immunizations were given and because of this the incidence of typhoid and smallpox was extremely low for those who were in the camps. Since the majority of the camp residents were poor blacks and whites, many were already on the border of malnutrition. The meals in the camps were supplemented with fresh vegetables and good quality protein. In addition, the Red Cross added a daily cake of powered yeast; the niacin in the yeast and the good diet helped to eliminate the pellagra.

Once the flood waters receded the Rockefeller Foundation helped to establish and fund health units in all of the affected counties.

Dr. Garrison and his small department helped in areas where they could. Due to the highway scandal that had been brewing for 10 years, the state was deep in debt. Despite this Garrison was able to convince Governor Martineau to put $23,000 of state money into the relief effort; this money was used as matching funds for the other agencies. Linnie Beauchamp was instrumental

in helping to recruit a large number of nurses to go into the affected areas and work. In North Little Rock, they set up a boxcar city to provide assistance for the refugees. At the beginning of the crisis, there were four fully staffed county health units around the state. As the camps were closed, 20 full-time units were established with the assistance of county and state government, U.S. Public Health Service, the Rockefeller Foundation and the Red Cross. Depending on the location, the Rockefeller Foundation provided from one-fourth to three-quarters toward the cost of these units.

Lest we paint too rosy a picture, it is important to remember that many of the camps were overcrowded and there was a significant difference between the camps for the African-Americans and the white sharecroppers. The land-owning planters expressed worry that if the black sharecroppers became too comfortable in the camps they would not return to work the fields in the summer and fall. Because of this, many of the black refugees were forced to leave the camps prematurely, at times even before the water had receded from their land. Once the sharecroppers left the camps, the planters became the dispensing agents for any aid. There were numerous reports that the returning sharecroppers had to pay for the aid as if buying from the company mercantile. Another important part of the Red Cross project included a resettlement plan where the displaced families were to get enough food for a month, seed for replanting, work animals if needed, food for their stock and temporary shelters. These resources were diverted as well and often were used to force the sharecroppers to work the land.

When the flood receded, large pockets of stagnant water remained with significant outbreaks of typhoid and malaria among those who had not been immunized. Because of the acute lack of garden plots, malnutrition, specifically pellagra, continued to be a major problem.

The last of the refugee camps closed on September 15, 1927 but the effect of the flood was felt for years.

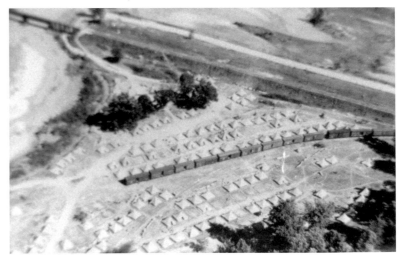

THE FORREST CITY CAMP IN ST. FRANCIS COUNTY HAD A RECORD NUMBER OF 15,850 DISPLACED PERSONS AT ITS HEIGHT. WHEN THEY ENTERED THE CAMP, EACH PERSON WAS REQUIRED TO RECEIVE AN IDENTIFICATION CARD TO OBTAIN CLOTHING AND FOOD. ALL WERE GIVEN SMALLPOX AND TYPHOID IMMUNIZATIONS.

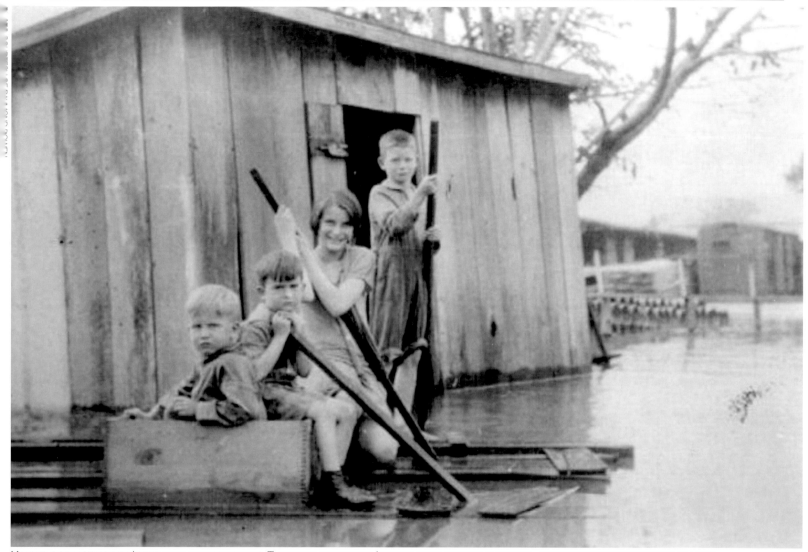

MANY FLOOD VICTIMS DIDN'T END UP IN REFUGEE CAMPS. THESE CHILDREN FROM AUGUSTA WERE USED TO FLOODING, JUST NOT THIS MUCH OR FOR THIS LONG.

THE DROUGHT OF 1930

The next health catastrophe to strike the state was the combined impact of the Drought of 1930-31 and the deepening economic Depression. The fall of Wall Street had little immediate effect of the general populace of Arkansas but when cotton prices bottomed out and it didn't rain for a year that got everyone's attention. With the exception of the large plantation farms in the Delta, most of the Arkansas farmers were small plot farms (60-70 acres) that survived primarily as subsistence farming. The American Dream for the people of rural Arkansas was 40 acres and a mule. The land was rich and if it rained enough, but not too much, the farmer and his family could survive. The days of rural electrification and significant irrigation were just around the corner but not yet a reality. When the rains stopped in 1930 and the land dried up, the corn, cotton and family gardens wilted and died. A mainstay of country life had always been wild game but those populations of animals had dwindled in the last two decades. When the drought hit and the fresh water sources dried up, the fish died and the wild game had to come out onto open stream beds and the banks of disappearing lakes for water. Many of the species such as bear, deer, turkey, coon, squirrel and rabbits that rural families depended on were quickly hunted to near extinction.

To men like Dr. Garrison, it quickly became obvious that the health of the public in Arkansas was about to take another hit. In the summer of 1930, he spoke to the Arkansas Drought Commission chaired by Harvey Couch, the head of Arkansas Power and Light. During his comments, he warned that unless early and significant relief measures were taken soon, widespread

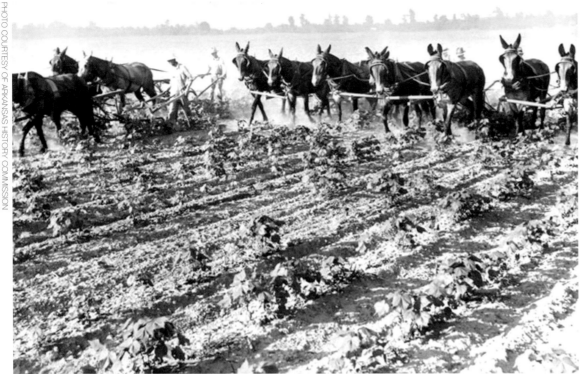

During the drought of 1930, eastern Arkansas planters expressed the view that "the only way to get Negros (and poor whites) to exert themselves as they should is to let them feel they will receive no help."

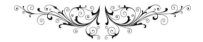

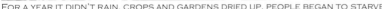

FOR A YEAR IT DIDN'T RAIN, CROPS AND GARDENS DRIED UP, PEOPLE BEGAN TO STARVE

starvation would soon be upon the state. Arguing against this view were the representatives of the eastern Arkansas planters who expressed the view that, "the only way to get Negros (and poor whites) to exert themselves as they should is to let them feel they will receive no help." The planters left the impression that they would take care of their own. On this occasion the Red Cross sided with the land owners and minimal aid was offered.

In December, after repeated pleas for assistance from around the state, Albert Evans, the Arkansas Red Cross director, made a survey of rural homes in Arkansas and found that there was no food and the planters were not providing any relief. Despite his report the national headquarters continued to stall.

The England "food riot" on January 3, 1931 got everyone's attention. A group of sharecroppers had failed to get any assistance because of a lack of Red Cross forms. After several attempts, they were joined by 500 black and white families and they all demanded the aid be released regardless of whether the proper forms were completed or not. Because of the negative national press caused by this event, Senator Thaddeus Caraway introduced an amendment to the $45 million Feed and Seed bill making its way through the Senate; the amendment would have provided $5 million in food aid. President Hoover viewed this amendment as dole and approached Judge John Payne of the National Red Cross to see if they could help. Payne assured Senator Caraway that his organization could raise the money that was

needed. Caraway's proposal was defeated.

Good to his word, Judge Payne began an aggressive fundraising campaign. In the first three months of 1931, the Red Cross fed 180,000 Arkansas families averting a health crisis of much larger proportion.

When Dr. Charles Garrison took over as the State Health Officer and Secretary of the State Board of Health in 1914, the organization was more of a dream than a reality; it was underfunded and its role undefined. Garrison commented that the public health services of Arkansas were "built on times of crisis such as floods, wars and droughts." He was devoted to and dearly loved by the nurses who worked with him. Most of these women shared his view of their role in the solving of the health problems of Arkansas and he stood up for them in times of crisis. He was well respected nationally and internationally. In 1924, he attended the International Health Conference in Copenhagen, Denmark and was recognized as one of those directors who had done the most with grants and funds available. In 1931, he was elected President of the State and Territorial Health Conference that met each year in Washington with the Surgeon General of the U. S. Public Health Service. A true believer; he was headstrong and independent; described by his foes as arrogant, rude and offensive, never shy about jumping into the middle of a controversy and calling a spade a spade. In an organization that often requires subtle political maneuvering as opposed to confrontation, Garrison occasionally was a fish out of water. He regularly fought with the more conservative members of the

state medical society and a few of the county medical societies over the role of the State Board of Health and the public health nurses. The gist of the argument revolved around preventive vs. curative care in patients who were able to pay. One recurring argument was that public health nurses were giving injections and other services to paying patients without physician supervision. The physicians made it clear they had no problem with the nurses giving injections to the poor without supervision. Despite a constant stream of this form of criticism Dr. Garrison and his allies went on about their business. It is clear that for the first 13 years of his

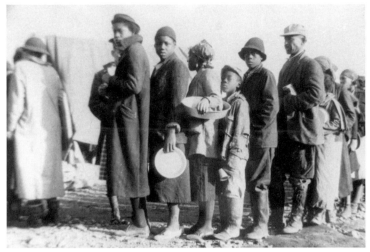

IN THE WINTER AND SPRING OF 1931, THE RED CROSS CAME TO THE RESCUE AGAIN, THIS TIME THE NEED WAS FOOD.

tenure he had a guardian angel in the person of Dr. Morgan Smith. Smith was the man who put together the coalition of forces that created the Board of Health, served briefly as the State Health Officer and then returned to his day job as the Dean of the University of Arkansas Medical School. He was a dominate figure in the Arkansas Medical Society for several decades. In 1927, he was lobbying the legislature to build a new building for the school and a hospital associated with the medical school. The legislature turned him down and, in fact, took money away from the school and re-allocated it to the prison system. On May 5, 1927, Morgan Smith resigned as Dean of the Medical School. Within months Charles Garrison was being forced to deal with a variety of problems. There were questions about his use of money and his ability to manage the day-to-day working of the Board of Health. In late 1928, Dr. Carl Michal, the lead physician with the U.S. Public Health Service in Arkansas, was granted an interview with Governor Parnell. A transcript of that meeting does not exist but clearly Dr. Michal was critical of Garrison and indicated that he felt that Garrison should be removed as the State Health Officer. Act 109 passed by the Arkansas General Assembly granted the Governor the authority to approve or disapprove the appointment of the State Health Officer. On May 12, 1929, the Board of Health sent out two letters. The first was sent to the U. S. Surgeon General requesting the immediate removal of Dr. Michal from his work in Arkansas. The second letter was to Governor Parnell re-affirming a new four year appointment of Dr. Garrison as State Health Officer. The governor approved of the appointment and this round was over.

By 1932, the State of Arkansas was nearing bankruptcy. Governor Marion Futrell of Greene County in East Arkansas was elected on a platform of cutting the budget. As opposed to his predecessor he was extremely conservative. One of his objectives was to cut all forms of state services, first on his list was higher education which he considered useless. Next on the list was public health, he refused to reappoint Dr. Garrison and instead appointed Dr. W. B. Grayson of Greene County, a former railroad surgeon who had no experience in public health. Grayson opposed mass immunization and other "socialist" programs. He made it clear that public health nurses were not to "practice medicine in any form or fashion," wholesale immunization was discouraged, and free clinics were to be discontinued unless organized by the county medical society. Reading the words attributed to Dr. Grayson sounded like they came out of the mouths of the most conservative members of the medical society.

After leaving the Board of Health, Dr. Garrison and his wife moved to Kentucky where he began taking refresher courses in preparation for a return to the private practice of medicine. During the time of his studies, he became ill with an undisclosed lung ailment and within two years was dead.

The Board of Health and public health system he left behind was a patchwork quilt of programs and funding that served the state well; but public health was about to go through a period of retrenchment.

Dr. W.B. Grayson of Greene County was a former railroad surgeon who had no experience in public health. He opposed mass immunization and other "socialist" programs. He made it clear that public health nurses were not to "practice medicine in any form or fashion," wholesale immunization was discouraged, and free clinics were to be discontinued unless organized by the county medical society.

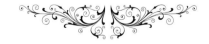

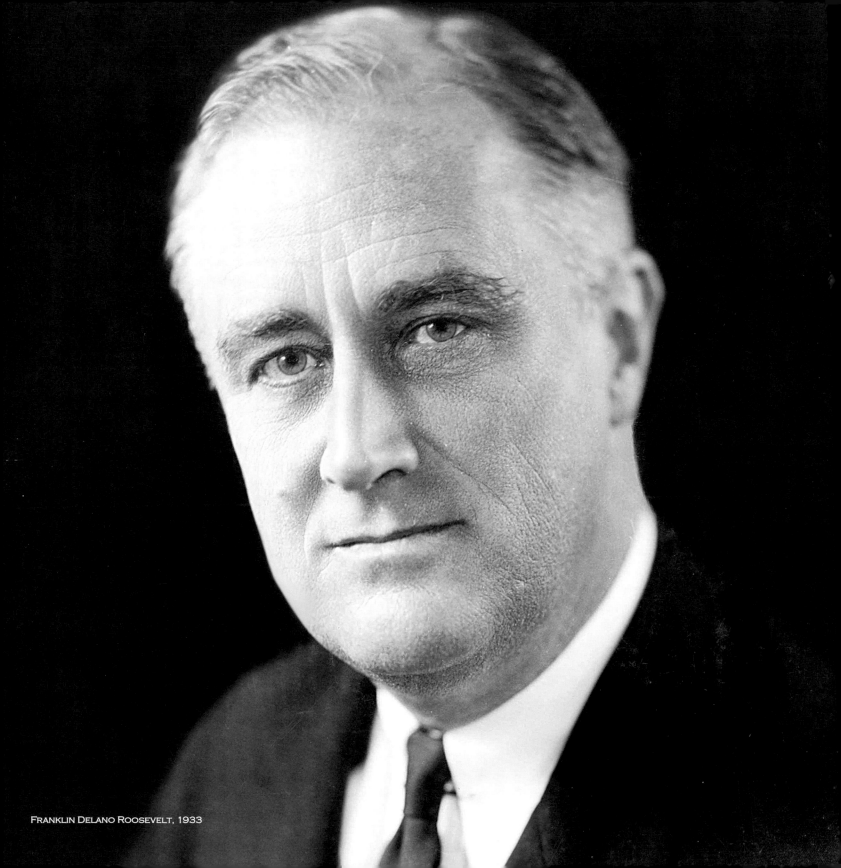

Franklin Delano Roosevelt, 1933

CHAPTER SIX
HAPPY DAYS ARE HERE AGAIN

In 1932, "Happy Days are Here Again," the campaign song for presidential hopeful Franklin Roosevelt, was not quite true in Arkansas but at least there was a glimmer of hope. Despite the Depression, the public's health was improving. Life expectancy from birth was beginning to rise; there were significant differences between urban and rural, rich and poor, white and black, but as the decade wore on, everyone's health rose to some extent. Infant mortality rates had begun to fall with the development of clean safe water and adequate sewer systems. A focus on pasteurization and improved milk quality had reduced the death rate from infant diarrhea. The health impact of rural electrification in the 1930s and 1940s is often overlooked but with population growth, the ability to develop electric-powered deep wells and remote lake water sources of potable water was increasingly important. Dependable functioning sewer systems that did not depend on dumping raw sewage into local rivers were slowly evolving. The in-home presence of refrigeration to prevent milk, meat and food spoilage allowed for improvements in year-round nutrition that were unheard of a generation before.

The above improvements with an increasing acceptance of immunization, understanding of the transmission of infectious disease, advancing knowledge of nutrition and its role in health were slowly changing the face of disease. Arkansas vital statistics prior to 1940 have a questionable degree of validity but as early as 1928 heart disease was listed as the number one cause of death in the population followed closely by tuberculosis. By 1940, heart disease was far and away the most common cause of death followed by cancer, stroke and in a distant fourth infectious disease including tuberculosis. These shifts reflect a population that was living well beyond infancy with many reaching old age. As late as 1940, tuberculosis continued to be the major killer of those between the age of 15 and 45 thus causing a great loss in productivity to the society.

When Roosevelt took office, the state had weathered the Flood of 1927, the Drought of 1930-31 and was now in the middle of the worst Depression in anyone's memory.

The 1920s had seen the beginnings of migration off of the farms by a significant number of the poor whites and now this was intensifying; many of these farmers looked toward the west coast for a better life. The African-American population had not participated in this migration in the 1920s but in the 1930s they began to leave the farm as well. Most of the blacks who left the farms did not leave the state; many simply moved to the edge of the nearest small towns or cities like Little Rock or Pine Bluff and lived in quickly constructed tarpaper shack communities. In the rural towns, many of these men and women ended up as day-laborers on the farms they had lived on just a year or two before; a significant number worked in cotton gins and sawmills. The housing, water and sanitation in these communities on the edge of the small rural towns was little different than what they had left in the country.

The Deep South, including the cotton growing parts of Arkansas, had been slow to mechanize but when the tractors did arrive it signaled the end of sharecropping and tenant farms. One tractor and one driver could do the work of 10 men each with a team of mules and at the end of the day the owner of the land didn't have to feed and house the man and his family.

The state of Arkansas was broke, public health and education funding were cut to the bone.

In 1931, just after the worst of the drought, there were 30 fully-staffed public health units across the state, by 1933 that number had dropped to 20. Part of this reduction in services had to do with a drop in support from the state, county and charity organizations and part was due to conflict between the private physician community and public health. Dr. Grayson, the new State Health officer, did not take a step without the approval of the Arkansas Medical Society.

"GRIT, GUMPTION AND GRACE"

Despite the lack of money and resources, the public health nurses were still out there; the Ladies in Blue covered the state.

In 1931, Ruby Odenbaugh Kinard was a young graduate nurse whose first assignment was Stone County. There was no such thing as electricity, no fresh vaccine, the roads were almost non-existent and typhoid was endemic. There is no written record to indicate if this was considered one of the fully-staffed health units but Ruby was the nurse, sanitarian, laboratory technician and secretary. There was one local physician who had signed on as the county health officer but he was not particularly helpful. Resistance to smallpox and typhoid immunization was strong and she spent a good deal of her time preaching the immunization gospel and organizing shot clinics. School attendance was low, so to reach many of the children who lived outside of Mountain View, she would take to her buggy or go out on horseback. She decided early on that the only liquid she could drink in the homes was coffee because it was boiled and did not provide a typhoid risk. Ruby sterilized her needles, syringes and other equipment with a Sterno heater. Children with developmental disabilities were common place and Ms. Beall at Children's Hospital in Little Rock took any children Ruby sent into Little Rock for care. She tells a delightful story of being broke and needing money for bandages and medicine for a sick child. It seems she had befriended a local bootlegger by going to see his sick children up in the hills and when he heard of her need, he provided her with the money she needed and continued to support her as long as she was in the community. For the next 43 years, she worked all over the state but always fondly remembered her time in the mountains.

In each community across the

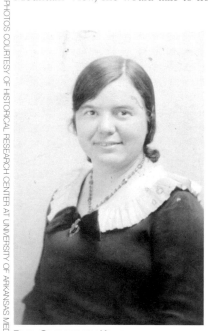

RUBY ODENBAUGH KINARD WAS A FRONTIER NURSE IN THE TRUEST SENSE OF THE WORD. SHE BEGAN HER PUBLIC HEALTH CAREER IN THE LATE 1930S IN STONE COUNTY AND FOR THE NEXT 43 YEARS WORKED ALL OVER THE STATE.

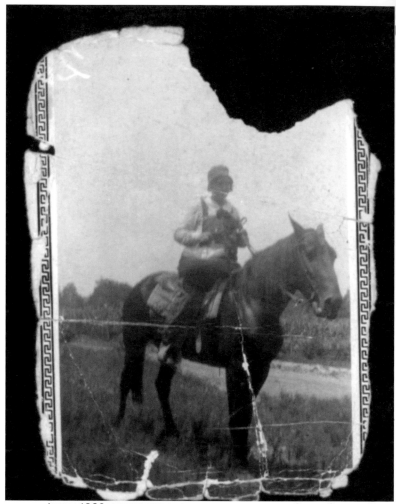

IN THE 1930S THERE WERE VERY FEW PAVED ROADS IN STONE COUNTY. RUBY ODENBAUGH KINARD SPENT A GREAT DEAL OF TIME ON HORSEBACK OR IN A BUGGY GOING TO SEE HER PATIENTS.

state, public health services varied considerably based on the needs of the community; Fort Smith and Pine Bluff are good examples. Because of its commercial activity, Fort Smith devoted a good deal of its effort to meat and food inspection with some involvement in treatment of the sick poor; they had almost no maternal and infant care or school screening programs. Pine Bluff, based on its population needs, spent far more time on treatment and prevention of communicable disease, home sanitation, child health screening and tuberculosis screening.

TUBERCULOSIS

It is hard to overestimate the effect of tuberculosis on the state of Arkansas; in 1928, it was the second largest reported cause of death in the state.

TB had a disproportionate impact on the black population of the state but there was no black sanatorium until 1931. Dr. George Ish, a prominent black physician in Little Rock, was active in black health care in central Arkansas for several decades and almost singlehandedly lobbied for and helped to create the McRae TB Sanatorium in Alexander, Arkansas. He was a member of the board of the institution from its inception until it closed in 1967.

The Booneville Sanatorium, founded in the first part of the century, was small compared to the need. With the backing of Leo Nyberg, a state representative from Phillips County and former TB patient at Boonville, the legislature passed a bill in 1930 that funded the construction of a large new hospital; the new facilities opened to patients in 1941.

Another of the state facilities that was showing signs of major problems was the Arkansas State Hospital. Founded in 1873 as the Arkansas Lunatic Asylum, by the mid-1920s it was full to overflowing. The legislature commissioned a study to look at the various options. In 1929, land was purchased in Saline County and, in 1934, the Benton Farm Colony of the State hospital was opened to patients.

THE NEW DEAL

Roosevelt's New Deal injected large amounts of aid and resources into Arkansas. Between 1933 and 1936, the Emergency Relief Administration provided $81 million to relieve distress and suffering due to unemployment in the state. In 1933, the State Relief Commission granted $24,000 to assist in maintaining county nurses and in providing vaccines. In November 1933, the Federal Relief Commission introduced a program called the Relief of Unemployed Needy Registered Nurses; in Arkansas, 350 nurses were hired and used for a variety of purposes. Of the nurses, 142 went to work directly for the State Board of Health and the rest did a variety of other tasks including first-aid instruction, operating first-aid stations, public education, school nursing and home sick care. Under the auspices of this program, 97,000 typhoid, 13,000 smallpox and 7,000 diphtheria immunizations were given. By 1935, the grants for health had risen to $611,000.

Under the same program, a number of resettlement camps were created, the most famous of these is the one at Dyess, Arkansas. These segregated camps were set up to provide a model community with modern sanitation and clean water. The Dyess camp was designed for 500 families with farm plots of 20 to 40 acres per family. Each of the camps had a small modern hospital and two physicians; much like in the Red Cross Camps, those who lived here were required to take smallpox and typhoid immunization. Malaria control was instituted.

In 1937, Johnny Cash was the 5-year-old son of a farmer in Dyess when the flood waters came a second time in 10 years. Years later he immortalized the Flood of 1937 in his song, "Five Feet High and Rising." That season the forces of nature conspired against the population of the Delta again. There are some estimates that the Flood of 1937 was actually worse than the Flood of 1927, the difference was that the levees on the Mississippi did not break. The other difference was there were simply not as many people living on the land and they were ready for it this time; the Red Cross, U.S. Public Health and the Arkansas Board of Health came to the rescue and

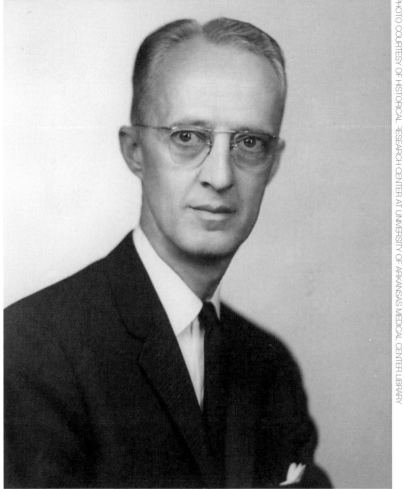

DR. J.T. HERRON JOINED THE STAFF OF THE ARKANSAS BOARD OF HEALTH IN 1939 AS A LOCAL HEALTH OFFICER. HE SERVED AS HEAD OF THE ARKANSAS BOARD OF HEALTH FROM 1951 TO 1971 AND LED THE ORGANIZATION THROUGH TIMES OF TURMOIL.

soon this too had passed.

The Social Security Act of 1935 was an attempt to reduce the dangers of modern life to the aged, the infirm, the poor, the unemployed, widows and fatherless children. Titles V and VI of this act had a significant impact on Arkansas health and disease going forward. By the end of the 1930s, the federal government provided almost two-thirds of the budget for the Arkansas State Board of Health. Title V of the act provided 13 percent of the budget through the U.S. Children's Bureau, Title VI provided for general public health and made up 35 percent of the budget and VD control amounted to 16 percent of the yearly expenditures. By the end of the 1930s, all 75 counties had full-time health services of some description. Fifteen counties had a full time physician, one or more public health nurses, a sanitarian and a clerk. Seventeen district health units combining three or more counties shared sanitarians and medical directors. As in the 1920s, county support made up

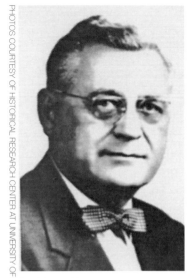

DR. EDGER EASLEY JOINED THE BOARD OF HEALTH IN 1939 AND WOULD SERVE UNTIL THE LATE 1970S. DURING WORLD WAR II HE ASSUMED THE ROLE OF STATE VD CONTROL OFFICER UNTIL HE WAS PROMOTED TO BE DR. HERRON'S SECOND IN COMMAND IN 1951.

the bulk of the funding for local health services. If very little money was forthcoming from the county, nursing service alone was provided.

It was around this time that two young physicians Dr. J.T. Herron and Dr. Edger Easley entered the picture of Arkansas's public health. These men hired into the health department during the depth of the Depression and maintained a presence until the mid-1970s helping to set the course of the agency.

Dr. J. T. Herron was born and raised in Little Rock, graduated from Central High in 1928, attended college at the University of Oklahoma and medical school at the University of Arkansas Medical School. Years later in a recorded interview, he recalled Dr. Grayson coming to his medical school class and talking about the exciting opportunities in public health brought on by the money from Social Security. Herron completed a residency in Internal Medicine at Scott-White Clinic in Temple, Texas and in 1939 returned to Little Rock where he made an attempt at private practice. He quickly discovered that private patients were far and few between. Again he was approached by Dr. Grayson and within two weeks he was a county health doctor with a salary of $250 a month and heading for the big city of Hamburg, Arkansas.

On arrival in the town of Hamburg, he was in for his trial by fire. Typhoid, diphtheria, malaria, syphilis and tuberculosis were prevalent and there hadn't been a public health doctor in at least a year. There were two other physicians in the community—an older regular physician and an eclectic physician; the two physicians didn't get along and they weren't the least bit happy he was there. Maternity and infant health care had been authorized and it was his job to get the pre-natal clinics going. VD clinics were being supported by the U. S. Public Health Service; the therapeutic agents used at that point were arsenic and bismuth, the treatments took 18 months of repeated IV therapy and they were painful. Many patients reacted to the therapy and never finished the treatment cycle. When interviewed in the 1970s, he stated that the saddest part was the children suffering from congenital syphilis; there were 10 to 20 of these children a year came through his clinic.

Dr. Herron's cohort was Dr. Edger Easley. He was born in Malvern and his family moved to Little Rock when he was seven. He attended the University of Arkansas Medical School and graduated in 1931. After medical school he joined the Navy where he was introduced to preventive medicine. In 1936 he fell on board his ship and had a significant head injury; in 1938 he was medically retired from the service and returned home. In 1939 he applied for and was accepted as a county health officer and within weeks he was heading for Texarkana. He arrived in the middle of a rain storm and was faced with a flooded office in the basement of the old courthouse. He immediately went to the office of the county judge and convinced the judge to accompany him to the flooded office; soon he had a non-flooding office in the new courthouse. After three months, he was moved to Arkadelphia. In 1940, the Board of Health sent him to Harvard to get a master's degree in Public Health with emphasis on syphilis control. When he returned World War II was in full swing and he became the VD Control Officer at Camp Robinson (formerly Camp Pike), after the war he became the State VD Control Officer.

During World War I venereal disease had become a major issue. A high percentage of the potential recruits were disqualified based on a positive blood test for syphilis; this continued to be true during World War II. At the beginning of World War II, Dr. J. T. Herron was doing induction physicals in Helena and 52 percent of the potential soldiers were turned down because of venereal disease. During World War I, a large center for VD control had been established in Hot Springs. In 1920, Dr. Oliver Clarence Wenger took over the clinic and made it a regional center for the diagnosis and treatment for syphilis. During the early 1930s, the numbers who presented to Wenger's clinic mushroomed. In 1933, the United States government created a Transients Bureau and a camp was opened on the eastern edge of Hot Springs near Gulpha Gorge. Camp Garrady acted as domicile for those on the road and for those in need of treatment for VD. Dr. Wenger reported that over the years, 80,000 men and women came through his camp and 36,000 needed treatment for syphilis. Wenger left in 1936 for an assignment in St. Louis. For a brief period of time an edict came down from the Board of Health that health department personal could diagnose syphilis but the patients must be sent to private physicians for treatment. It is tempting to think that this was another issue where the State Health Officer, Dr. Grayson, bowed to the medical society but it is more likely in this instance that

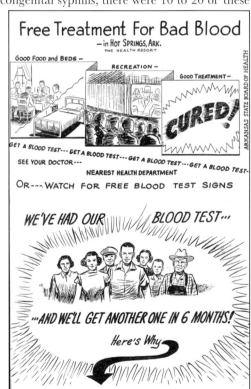

IN THE DAYS PRIOR TO PENICILLIN, SYPHILIS AND GONORRHEA WERE MAJOR PROBLEMS, ESPECIALLY AMONG THE BLACK POPULATION. DR. HERRON WAS DOING INDUCTION PHYSICALS IN HELENA AT THE BEGINNING OF WORLD WAR II AND 52 PERCENT OF THE INDUCTEES WERE TURNED DOWN BECAUSE OF VD.

there was simply no money. In less than a year, the U. S. Public Health Service began providing funds for the treatment of VD and the public health facilities were back in the business of treating. In addition to treating sick patients, the U. S. Public Health Service provided a VD truck that traveled from town to town. Rapid treatment regimens were created that allowed VD patients to be treated for a shorter period of time and released; this dramatically improved the compliance and successful completion of therapy. Dr. Easley commented in an interview in the 1970s that they often had a deal with the judges in the counties where they worked. It seems that significant numbers of the patients were also prisoners in the local jail or faced charges in the local courts. If a syphilis carrier followed through on treatment to the finish, any charges held outstanding would be dismissed. In six to eight years, penicillin became available making most of this unnecessary.

WORLD WAR II

As the war approached, many of the resources devoted to health were diverted to the military buildup. The economic problems of the Depression had encouraged many young physicians and nurses to go into public health. During the war, large numbers of these young professionals left for military service and never returned to public health. Prosperity after the war enticed many of the medical workers out of public health into private practice and research; this paucity of professionals plagued the Arkansas Board of Health for the next two decades.

The Second World War dramatically reduced unemployment in Arkansas with the emergence of two large army bases, Camp Robinson in Little Rock and Fort Chaffee in Fort Smith and six ordnance plants producing fuses, bombs and detonators. Since a large percentage of the able bodied young men were off at war, many of those employed were young women. As opposed to farm work most of these new jobs were well paid and highly valued. Saline County saw a boom with the building of a large aluminum production facility in the town of Bauxite. The oil industry surrounding El Dorado produced as much as 30 million barrels a year during the war years.

During the war, there were 23,000 German and Italian prisoners of war spotted around Arkansas on military and branch camps. There were 16,000 Japanese-Americans in two camp towns in the Delta: Rohwer and Jerome. The health care for the German and Italian soldiers was provided by the U.S. Army and the U.S. Public Health Service provided services for the Japanese. The Public Health Service and the U.S. Army insisted that those working on the camps have their immunizations; they demanded good clean water systems, adequate sewers, clean food and milk. In each of the facilities created for the war effort, the same effort was put into the surrounding communities as was done during World War I at Camp Pike and Arkansas's basic infrastructure benefited.

Despite the malaria prevention knowledge accumulated in the previous 40 years there were still several thousand cases of malaria reported each year in the state of Arkansas. In 1944, DDT was made available by the U.S. Army for wide distribution. All of the areas surrounding federal facilities were sprayed; mosquitoes and malaria were dramatically reduced. In addition, typhus, also known as "jail fever" because of its propensity to be associated with filth, rats and fleas was added to the list of diseases they pursued. The primary strategy was to kill off the rats and improve trash control. At one point a survey of captured rats in Little Rock and North Little Rock revealed 25 percent tested positive for typhus. One promotion provided a free ticket to the movies for every rat tail turned in.

After the war, the U.S. Public Health Service, in conjunction with the State Board of Health, began spraying thousands of homes every year with DDT. By 1951, there were no reported cases of malaria or typhus in the state. The World War II Malaria Control program centered in Atlanta eventually evolved into the Communicable Diseases Center or as we know it today CDC.

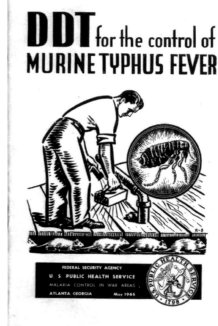

PHOTO COURTESY OF HISTORICAL RESEARCH CENTER AT UNIVERSITY OF ARKANSAS MEDICAL CENTER LIBRARY

A SURVEY OF RAT POPULATIONS IN LITTLE ROCK AND NORTH LITTLE ROCK DEMONSTRATED THAT 25 PERCENT WERE INFECTED WITH TYPHUS. ONE PROMOTION PROVIDED A FREE TICKET TO THE MOVIES FOR EVERY RAT TAIL TURNED IN.

MATERNAL, INFANT AND MIDWIVES

In the early part of the war, Dr. J.T. Herron served as the County Health Doctor in Helena in Phillips County. In 1943 he was moved to Little Rock to become the Director of Health Services. One of his principal jobs during this phase of his career was to administer the Emergency Maternal and Infant Care program. EMIC was a program funded by the federal government to make sure that the wives and small children of servicemen rank of E-5 (sergeant) and below were cared for during pregnancy and the first year of life. At the beginning of the war, less than 50 percent of white and 10 percent of black women in Arkansas had their children in a hospital. Almost immediately Herron had 100-200 applications for service a day. Theoretically the system was to be color blind; however, since the state's hospital beds were strictly segregated and there were very few black maturity beds available, most of the resources went to the white applicants. The program was well received except by the doctors of the state. The notes of Board of Health meetings and the various reports of the more conservative members of the Arkansas Medical Society indicate that the physicians had concerns that this attempt to provide services to the poor would broaden and interfere with their practice of medicine—taking away potentially paying patients. Despite the fact that the national program continued for a good while after the war, Arkansas was

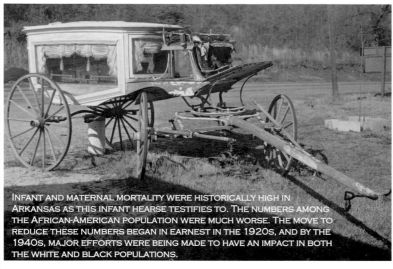

INFANT AND MATERNAL MORTALITY WERE HISTORICALLY HIGH IN ARKANSAS AS THIS INFANT HEARSE TESTIFIES TO. THE NUMBERS AMONG THE AFRICAN-AMERICAN POPULATION WERE MUCH WORSE. THE MOVE TO REDUCE THESE NUMBERS BEGAN IN EARNEST IN THE 1920S, AND BY THE 1940S, MAJOR EFFORTS WERE BEING MADE TO HAVE AN IMPACT IN BOTH THE WHITE AND BLACK POPULATIONS.

one of the first to withdraw from the services.

The other thorny subject was the use of midwives especially among the black population. A survey conducted in 1926 revealed that there were 4,000 midwives in the state. Under the Sheppard-Towner Act, many of these women received some instruction from the Board of Health. As late as 1940, 80 percent of black births were attended by a midwife in the home whereas less than 10 percent of white births utilized a midwife. In the late 1930s, Dr. Francis Rothert, formerly of the U.S. Children's Bureau, joined the Arkansas Board of Health as head of Maternity and Infant Care. She was involved in a number of programs aimed at improving newborn and infant care including the first premature baby program in the state. The State Board of Health purchased a number of incubator bassinettes that were loaned to families of low birth weight babies. Rothert worked closely with Jeff Farris Sr. at Arkansas Teachers College in Conway to educate teachers and nurses for improvements in school health. She helped to establish a home care program for Premature Low Birth Weight babies in Jefferson County. The thorniest issue she dealt with was the subject of educating the black midwives. The infant mortality rate for black children was almost twice that of whites. A good part of the problem could be laid at the feet of poverty and malnutrition, but some of the data pointed to the black midwives. Many of the black "granny" midwives were between ages 60 to 80, illiterate and had no formal training. The infant mortality and incidence of puerperal death where these midwives attended the birth were very high. As with many country physicians, cleanliness and hand washing were not part of their normal routine. Dr. Rothert related that one country physician in Arkansas proudly insisted that he always washed his hands after the delivery. The Arkansas Medical Society had turned a blind eye to the problem for the last century in great part because it was seen as a "negro" problem. The society was hesitate to see the Board of Health getting into the business of teaching and certifying the midwives because to them this was a slippery slope that would lead to more programs like the government sponsored Maternal and Infant Aid during the war. After making several impractical suggestions they acquiesced for the board to provide instruction and licensing of the midwives.

In the summer of 1945, Dr. Rothert appointed Mamie Hale, a young black Tuskegee trained Nurse-Midwife, to develop and conduct education programs and supervise the black midwives of the state. Over a five year period, Ms. Hale moved across the state with a religious fervor. Since many of her students were illiterate, the instructions were simple, clear and straightforward. She emphasized hand washing and cleanliness. The midwives were encouraged not to wear rubber gloves and not to do an internal exam. Though the admonition against gloves may seem counterintuitive the logic was: if they did not wear gloves they would be less inclined to do internal exams and less likely to create problems with infection. The midwives were instructed in the signs of significant problems and the steps to be taken when they occurred. Routine care of the newborn and newborn resuscitation were major parts of their training.

When the training was complete, they were treated to an elaborate graduation ceremony and licensed for one year; staying certified required yearly attendance to refresher courses.

When the program began there were 1,403 midwives identified in the state and by 1950 that number had dropped to 960. Many of the older midwives simply retired rather than go through the training. Seventy-five percent of all midwife deliveries were done by those with state permits.

In 1952, the Board of Health passed a regulation that allowed for the prosecution of violators of the permitting process. The State Board of Health eventually brought charges against eight habitual offenders on charges varying from practicing without a permit to doing abortions.

A continuing problem was the lack of sufficient physician-based obstetrics to help with complicated problems. In 1948, the University of Arkansas Medical School utilized senior medical students under the supervision of the State Board of Health to man rural obstetric clinic around the state and act as a referral source for the midwives.

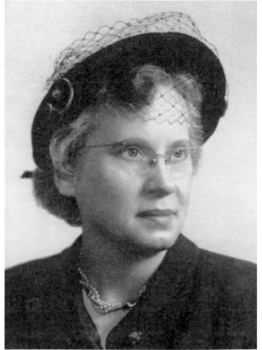

DR. FRANCIS ROTHERT WAS A DEDICATED PEDIATRICIAN WHO HELPED TO GUIDE THE ARKANSAS BOARD OF HEALTH MATERNAL AND INFANT HEALTH PROGRAM FOR 20-PLUS YEARS.

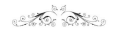

Dr. Rothert related that one country physician in Arkansas proudly insisted that hc always washed his hands "after the delivery."

The overall numbers of maternal and infant deaths did improve, however, by1954 the black mother and child were still three times as likely to have serious complication surrounding the time of birth as were white mothers.

It would take several decades and the desegregation of facilities and services before any real progress would be made in the gap between blacks and whites.

POLITICS RAISES ITS HEAD, AGAIN

From its inception, the operations of the State Board of Health have been involved in the machinations of politics. Regulations promulgated by the department have often been met with an immediate appeal to the legislature on the part of an affected business groups. The canning industry and the meat packing industry attempted a number of end runs in the 1950s and 1960s. And it wasn't just industry, the Arkansas Medical Society was never hesitant to politically undermine and influence regulations or decisions they found distasteful. In January 1941, the Board of Health made the judgment not to get involved in contraception; in April 1941, the Arkansas Medical Society suggested that the board get involved in contraception for those who could not pay and they did.

Like most governors before and since, Governor Homer Adkins (1941-1945) believed strongly in political patronage. In his first year in office, he placed a number of friends and political cronies in the Bureau of Vital Statistics. By February 1943, there was a crisis in the bureau; the registrations of birth and death certificates were not getting recorded. There are estimates of several thousand piled around on desks in the office waiting to be processed. When the Board learned of the problem they contacted the governor through Dr. Grayson and asked for his assistance in putting the bureau back on a sound footing. The governor came to the next board meeting and after a heated encounter acceded to their request. In return he wanted several of his appointees to be left in place for a time until he could find an appropriate place for them. There is no written record of what happened over the next several months but at the July meeting of the board, the governor was present again and this time, very angry, demanding the firing of Dr. Grayson. In short order the Board fired Dr. Grayson and appointed Dr. T.T. Ross, an apolitical physician, who stayed at the post until 1951. Despite his firing, Dr. Grayson assumed the role of liaison with the Arkansas Medical Society for several years, reporting to them on the activities of the board. There are no records that indicate whether this pleased or displeased the governor.

CHANGE IS AT HAND

The end of World War II marked another dramatic change for the future of health and disease in Arkansas and the United States. The mass production of sulfa drugs and penicillin transformed the practice of medicine and public health. X-ray units and EKG machines became common place in physician's offices. House calls slowly gave way to office calls. In rural communities, small doctor's hospitals were slowly replaced by community hospitals. Heart disease, cancer and stroke replaced infectious disease as the major killers in American society.

Public health was forced to take a second and third look at their priorities. A large number of non-farm light industrial companies, such as shoe and garment factories, were established after the war as the poultry industry in northwest Arkansas also began a major expansion. With the shift away from traditional farm labor, the Board of Health created the Division of Industrial Hygiene aimed at formulating regulations to ensure safety in the work site.

The emergence of the chronic diseases of aging brought a number of changes. In 1946, an Arkansas Cancer Commission was established to monitor the incidence and distribution of various forms of cancer. In October 1946, an initiative for Mental Health Hygiene was launched. In 1950 a Heart Disease program was begun in conjunction with the University of Arkansas Medical Center. The Cancer Commission, Heart Disease program and the continued focus on Tuberculosis were paired with volunteer national and local societies—the American Cancer Society, the American Heart Association and the American Lung Association. Each of these organizations helped to develop the constituencies for research and preventive health strategies that framed the approaches to chronic disease in the second half of the 20th century.

In 1948, the Framingham Heart Study began in the small town of Framingham, Massachusetts. It started with a population of 5,000 healthy subjects between the ages of 30 and 60. In 2013 the study is still ongoing and is now into its third generation of these families. Before the advent of this study, heart disease, hypertension and stroke were considered simply a consequence of growing older. In this study the assumption was made that these diseases could be influenced by the way one lives their life and the surroundings where they live. This is the study that coined the phrase risk factors for disease. By the early 1960s, they began publishing the first of their studies and changed the way we view health and disease in modern society.

The Hill-Burton Act of 1946 had an immediate impact on the health and disease patterns in Arkansas. The U.S. Public Health made it clear as early as 1943 that the lack of available medical resources and facilities in the United States was a stumbling block to improving the health of this country especially among the poor. The purpose of the Act was to create a minimum of 4.5 hospital beds/1,000 citizens by providing grants-in-aid to communities across the country through an agency of state government; this program was later expanded to include long-term care facilities.

The Arkansas State Board of Health was the agency that handled these funds. In 1945, Dr. J.T. Herron did a statewide survey looking at what was available and the adequacy of those facilities. The results were as expected.

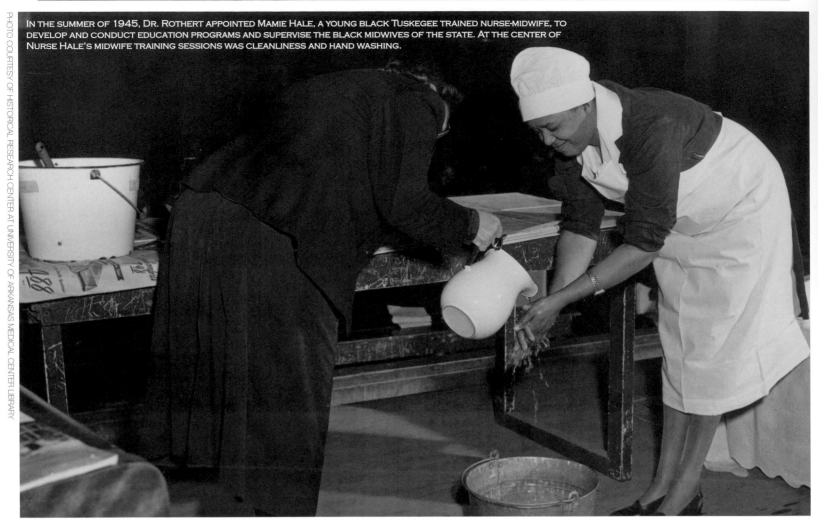

IN THE SUMMER OF 1945, DR. ROTHERT APPOINTED MAMIE HALE, A YOUNG BLACK TUSKEGEE TRAINED NURSE-MIDWIFE, TO DEVELOP AND CONDUCT EDUCATION PROGRAMS AND SUPERVISE THE BLACK MIDWIVES OF THE STATE. AT THE CENTER OF NURSE HALE'S MIDWIFE TRAINING SESSIONS WAS CLEANLINESS AND HAND WASHING.

Several of the larger communities such as Little Rock and Fort Smith had long established hospitals that functioned as primary care centers for the cities and tertiary referral care for the rest of the state. Most small towns were served by physician hospitals that began as lying-in hospitals—several rooms attached to the doctor's office for use in obstetrics. The quality of care provided in these facilities was often very poor. Another issue was the strict segregation of services. Effectively there were a small number of facilities that cared for the black population; because of this a "separate-but-equal" clause was written into the Hill-Burton Act. In the end there were only 10 facilities built in the entire of the United States to fulfill this requirement, one in Arkansas.

Officially the AMA and the Arkansas Medical Society did not oppose this act but segments of the medical community who owned their own facilities and saw them as profit centers lobbied against these hospitals, raising the specter of state medicine and socialism.

Part of the requirement to receive funding was that the hospital provided care for low-income/non-paying patients. The first hospital built with this money in Arkansas was Crittenden Memorial Hospital in West Memphis. It was completed in 1951 and it did provide beds for blacks and whites in segregated wards.

Eventually Hill-Burton funds were used to construct 350 projects including hospitals, nursing homes and health clinics in Arkansas. This provided the beginnings of the infrastructure for Arkansas health care for the last half of the 20th century.

FOOD, DRUGS AND THE CANNING INDUSTRY

In 1938, the Congress updated the Pure Food and Drug Act of 1906 with the passage of the Food, Drug and Cosmetic Act; the national legislation only related to products that crossed state lines. In 1939, the state of Arkansas followed that up with its own complementary law and the formation of the Division of Food and Drug Control within the State Board of Health. As with many of the commissions and divisions created during this timeframe, almost no state or local funding was forthcoming. It wasn't until after the war that the division had the resources to begin carrying out its mission. After World War II, Harold Austin, a Kansas pharmacist, and two inspectors were hired and began pursuing problems in the meat packing and the canning industry. A legitimate and reputable canning industry had existed in Arkansas for several decades; however the Depression and World War II saw the emergence of several hundred "shade tree" factories most of which were no more than a barn or a lean-to; most had no sanitary facilities, their water source was often a stream that ran near the barn and they paid very little attention to the product they canned. This came to a head in 1950 with a worm infestation in the locally raised spinach crop. The reputable canners simply canned no spinach and encouraged the rest to follow suit. When many of the small operators continued to package their product, the canner's cooperative notified Austin and his inspectors. Soon the inspectors quarantined large parts of the canned products and called in the federal inspectors. In an attempt to do an end-run the canners went to the legislature and were in the process of having a bill passed that would have eliminated the power of the Board of Health. Dr. Ross, Harold Austin, the federal inspectors and the Arkansas Valley Canning Association, representing the larger canners, lined up

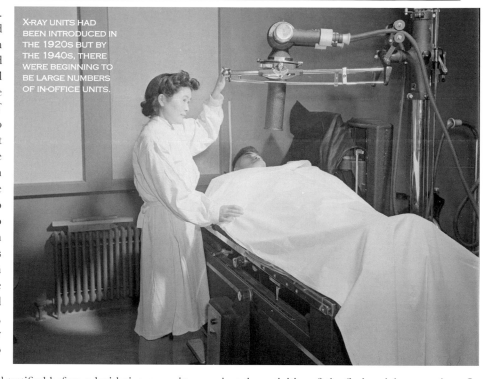

X-RAY UNITS HAD BEEN INTRODUCED IN THE 1920S BUT BY THE 1940S, THERE WERE BEGINNING TO BE LARGE NUMBERS OF IN-OFFICE UNITS.

and testified before a legislative committee against the activities of the fly-by-night operations. In the end no legislative action was taken and the Food and Drug Division was well established even if they were not well funded.

In Arkansas the 1950s was dominated by the issue of race and most of the news was unpleasant. Many of the state's white politicians used race baiting as a way to get elected. In 1948 two events occurred that would show the path that desegregation should ideally have taken. In February, Silas Hunt a black World War II veteran, met with Dr. Robert A. Leflar, dean of the University of Arkansas Law School, and applied for admission to the law school. Leflar lobbied the administration of the university and then the governor; in the end Hunt was admitted. After his first year of classes, young Mr. Hunt became quite ill and in April 1949 died of tuberculosis. Just a few short months after Silas Hunt was accepted to law school at the University of Arkansas, Edith Irby was accepted to the University of Arkansas Medical School and began classes. Born and raised in rural Arkansas, she was a good student and had been accepted to a number of medical schools out of state but she wanted to attend school in Arkansas. She became the first African-American to attend medical school in Arkansas. In a class of 91 students, she was the only black and one of only three women. After she completed her education, she practiced in Hot Springs for several years and then moved to Houston where she completed a residency in Internal Medicine. She and her husband settled in Houston where she spent the rest of her professional life developing facilities to help deal with the problems of the poor and especially the poor blacks of that city.

In June 1950, the Korean War began and, as with other wars, federal funds for public health were slashed. In states like Arkansas that depended heavily on federal aid, this would have a major impact. Dr. Tom Ross was not in good health and in 1951 made the decision to step down as the State Health Officer. Dr. J.T. Herron took over as State Health Officer and immediately named Dr. Edgar Easley as his Assistant and Deputy Director of Local Health Services. For the next 21 years, these two men would the set the course of public health in Arkansas.

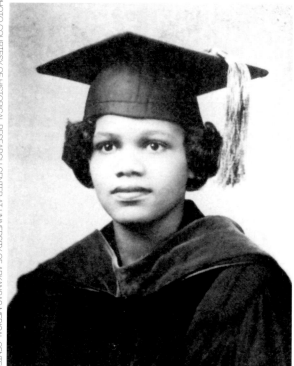

EDITH IRBY WAS THE FIRST AFRICAN-AMERICAN TO BE ADMITTED TO THE UNIVERSITY OF ARKANSAS MEDICAL SCHOOL.

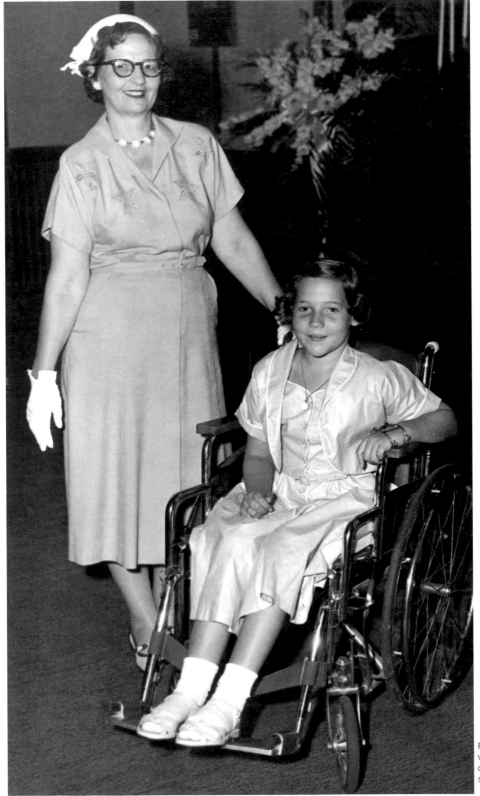

POLIOMYELITIS STRUCK
WITHOUT WARNING,
CHANGING THE LIVES OF
SMALL CHILDREN FOREVER.

CHAPTER SEVEN
TURMOIL AND CHANGE

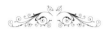

"We all feared polio. Everyone talked about it. It was December 22, 1950 and I was seven years old. My sister and I were going to dance in the Riggs Dance recital. As part of the show each of us would go to the front of the stage, they would pull the curtain aside and we would curtsey, then the curtain would shut. After we all did our curtsey, then the curtain would open again and we would all do our dance. When I began to curtsey, I fell to the floor. My left leg just gave way. The audience laughed and I was carried off the stage. My sister and mother thought I was mad and embarrassed and just didn't want to dance, but I wasn't. By the next morning I couldn't stand. My mother called Dr. Ashby, he looked me over and said, 'This girl has polio. We have to get her to the University Medical Center now.' I began to cry because I knew at that instant that the life I had dreamed of had changed and I would never be the same again."

Marilyn Cox

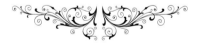

These are the memories of Marilyn Cox of Benton, Arkansas. Her mother was Mary Cox, the Public Health nurse for Saline County from 1946-1971. For the next 12 years her mother and father spent every cent they could make and every minute of time they had making sure that this young lady survived. Despite the permanent paralysis of her legs and back and partial paralysis of arms and hands, she went on to lead a pretty normal life. She ended up with a master's degree in psychology and worked for 25 years helping other disabled adults with rehabilitation.

Poliomyelitis, a viral illness, also called polio or infantile paralysis, made its first appearance in the United States in 1894 in Vermont. Polio is a devastating illness that strikes primarily children, presenting with high fever, severe headaches, back and leg pain, vomiting and irritability. A small number of cases progress to infection of the central nervous system with destruction of the motor nerves supplying the muscles, the result is paralysis. Severe infections may extend into the brain causing apnea and requiring the need of an iron lung.

Prior to 1937, Arkansas reported only sporadic cases of polio. In the summer of 1937, an epidemic was reported across the South. In July and August, Arkansas reported 344 cases with 13 deaths; as with the flu in 1918, there was little that could be done except for the old standbys of quarantine and supportive care.

The Crippled Children's Division of the State Department of Welfare was formed and staffed by Dr. Francis Rothert of the State Board of Health. The resources she had were meager but with the help of Arkansas Children's Hospital and local private surgeons, they patched together a program to deal with these paralyzed children. Over the next few years, Arkansas Children's Hospital and the Army-Navy Hospital in Hot Springs provided therapy for those suffering from the ravages of polio.

The next major polio outbreak occurred in the summer of 1949. Dr. Davis Fitzhugh, who eventually became the Deputy Director of the Arkansas Health Department, was a senior medical student when the first cases started to trickle in. Soon the trickle turned to a flood and every available bed was full at the University Medical Center, Baptist Hospital and St. Vincent's. At one point the women's mess hall at the University Medical Center was full of iron lungs breathing for these small children. In all there were 992 cases

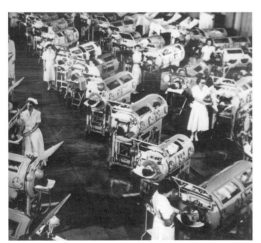

FOR DECADES THERE HAD BEEN MINOR EPIDEMICS OF POLIO IN THE UNITED STATES. IN 1949 IT HIT WITH A VENGEANCE. THE HOSPITALS IN CENTRAL ARKANSAS WERE FULL OF SICK CHILDREN, MANY NEEDING THE ASSISTANCE OF AN IRON LUNG.

requiring some form of intensive care in the state. Basil O'Conner, the head of the National Foundation for Infantile Paralysis, visited the state and helped to provide the equipment and supplies necessary to care for the patients.

In 1950, the Arkansas Polio Planning Committee was formed under the leadership of Dr. Ross and Dr. Herron of the Board of Health and Dr. Francis Rothert of the Crippled Children's Division of the Department of Welfare. Also included were representatives of the hospitals of Central Arkansas, the Red Cross and the National Foundation for Infantile Paralysis (NPIF). Several retired public health nurses, among them Linnie Beauchamp and Mary Emma Smith, were active in helping to develop training programs for nurses in dealing with polio patients.

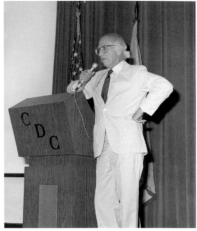

JONAS SALK, DEVELOPER OF THE POLIO VACCINE.

Since 1934 researchers had been working on a vaccine for polio. By 1950 Jonas Salk, a researcher funded by the NFIP, found what he thought might be the answer: a killed vaccine of poliovirus. One of Salk's leading critics was Albert Sabin who was working on a live-attenuated vaccine; he was convinced that Salk's vaccine would be too weak.

By early 1953, Mr. O'Conner of the NFIP and Dr. Salk began making plans for a mass randomized study to show the efficacy and safety of the vaccine. By the spring of 1954 they were ready. The plan was to vaccinate 1.8 million children nationwide. In Arkansas, five counties with 5,029 grade school children were vaccinated with the Salk vaccine; the counties included were Craighead, Jefferson, Mississippi, Pulaski and Sebastian. The initial numbers would have been larger had it not been for a radio broadcast by Walter Winchell where he opined that the new vaccine might be a killer; that it had been shown to contain live virus and had killed several monkeys. Despite the public assurance of a blue-ribbon panel of virologists that the vaccine was safe, estimates are that the participation rates were down about 40 percent in the states of Michigan, Arkansas and Ohio. On April 26, 1954, Randy Kerr of McLean, Virginia received the first injection and by the end of June, 626,779 children had received two of the series of three inoculations.

On April 12, 1955, the first results of the study were announced—against the three common forms of the polio virus the vaccine was 70-100% effective with limited reactions. The vaccine was immediately licensed for national distribution and the impact was dramatic: In 1955, there were 29,000 cases of polio in the United States and by 1957 only 5,900. There were a small number of children who developed forms of polio but overall the probabilities of side effects were very low.

Once the initial study was complete and results were in, the next question was: where would the money come from to immunize all of the children in the United States? Congress was quick to answer that question and on August 12, 1955, President Eisenhower signed into law the Polio Vaccination Law of 1955 which provided $90 million for the purchase and distribution of the Salk polio vaccine for children across the nation.

In Arkansas, there were 202,000 children ages five to nine who were eligible for the series of three immunizations. The next problem was how to organize for the management of such a large project. The State Polio Planning Committee mandated that each county form its own planning committee to include public health officials, county medical society physicians, pharmacists, school administrators and lay members. Ninety percent of the vaccine available was purchased by the federal government and distributed by the National Public Health Service and the NFIP. Ten percent of the vaccine was available through commercial sources and given by physicians in their offices. In a few counties the physicians created an obstacle because of their insistence on being present for each immunization and being paid for each injection. In March 1956, the physicians went on record as being opposed to the government vaccine act as passed by Congress. Despite these obstacles and in part because of the persistence of Dr. Herron and his committee, 87,832 were vaccinated in 1955; most were done in mass clinics held in schools.

In the late spring of 1955, one glitch occurred that created shortages for the summer. It was discovered that vaccine manufactured by Cutter Laboratories was causing problems with children in Illinois and California. It turned out that some of the vaccine did make it to the distribution chain in Arkansas but none was ever given.

Despite objections from the Medical society, the original Federal Vaccine Act was extended and the government provided vaccine from 1955 to 1959. For three years the rates of polio dropped and by 1957 the polio rate was at a very low level. In 1959, there was a dramatic increase in polio especially across the South. The Governor of Arkansas declared an emergency and allocated $50,000 for the care of children ill with polio. This time the distribution of illness fell heaviest on poor African-American children. Eighty-eight percent of those with polio had had either no vaccination or less than the full series of three injections and 87 percent of the less-than-five age group had either not been vaccinated or their series was incomplete.

In 1960, Dr. Herron commented in a report to the Arkansas Medical Society, "There is no provision for furnishing polio vaccine through the State Health Department. This is regrettable, since all surveys have definitely indicated that the low socio-economic groups have received the least polio protection at all age levels."

While the Salk vaccine project had been carried out, Albert Sabin was working on an oral attenuated-virus vaccine that would more closely mimic the active polio virus thereby producing better immunity. By 1957 he was ready for human trials and by 1962 his oral vaccine was licensed. The vaccine was given on a sugar cube and soon became the choice for mass inoculations; it was cheaper to make and easier to take than Salk's injectable vaccine.

In October 1962, the Congress passed a second Vaccination Assistance Act and money began to flow into the states to create a campaign of mass immunization. Prior to these mass immunization clinics sampling surveys done across Arkansas revealed inadequate immunization among all age groups and all races.

On a series of Sabin Sundays in 1963, tens of thousands of Arkansans were immunized with a small amount of oral vaccine on a sugar cube. Dr. Roger Bost, a Fort Smith physician and Chairman of the American Medical Society polio committee, commented on the mass sugar cube inoculations: "The incidence of polio throughout the country, and in Arkansas, went to virtually zero. Polio became a disease of the past."

A DEADLY TORNADO

Late in the evening March 21, 1952 Arkansas suffered its most deadly storm. The storm spawned tornadoes across the southern United States with 209 total deaths, 112 of which were in Arkansas. Worst hit were the

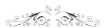

In 1960, Dr. Herron commented in a report to the Arkansas Medical Society, "There is no provision for furnishing polio vaccine through the State Health Department. This is regrettable, since all surveys have definitely indicated that the low socio-economic groups have received the least polio protection at all age levels."

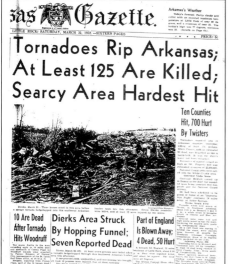

LATE IN THE EVENING ON MARCH 21, 1952, ARKANSAS SUFFERED ITS MOST DEADLY STORM. THE STORM SPAWNED TORNADOES ACROSS THE SOUTHERN UNITED STATES WITH 209 TOTAL DEATHS, 112 OF WHICH WERE IN ARKANSAS. IN JUDSONIA ALONE, 50 PEOPLE DIED.

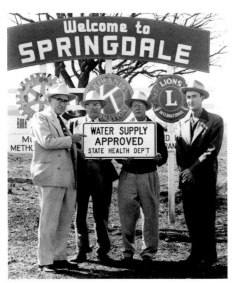

GLEN KELLOGG AND E.C. SPRATT HELPED TO RE-ESTABLISH WATER AND SANITATION SERVICES TO THE STORM STRICKEN AREA.

small towns of Judsonia in White County and Cotton Plant in Woodruff County. Cotton Plant suffered 20 deaths and Judsonia 50. Glen Kellogg was a young sanitary engineer who had been hired by the Board of Health in 1947. He started as an Assistant District Engineer and eventually worked his way up to Chief Engineer for the state. On the night of March 21, he and a group of his cohorts were notified by Dr. Herron of the potential catastrophe they had on their hands. They marshaled their small forces and made their way to Judsonia. By all estimates Kellogg was a man who had a command presence; quickly, he evaluated the situation, called his boss and informed him of the destruction. It turned out that 385 homes had been destroyed and another 560 had major damage; the power, water and sewer systems were completely incapacitated.

By the next morning, Kellogg and his crew had set to work re-establishing clean water and sewage control. The National Guard, Public Health Nurses and Red Cross were soon on the ground aiding the victims. This was the first Arkansas natural disaster where most of the resources needed to deal with a major crisis were present on the ground and organized to prevent other problems.

Glen Kellogg served as the Chief Sanitary Engineer for the State from 1955 to 1978. Like Zach Bair before him, he was instrumental in upgrading the water and sewer systems in the state. He became an early champion for mandatory water licensing and buffer zones around all water sources. By 1973, 83 percent of the state's population was served by public water systems and 54 percent had public sewer systems. He was behind the Water Supply Approved Signs that towns and cities were allowed to erect to distinguish particular water supplies for standards of excellence. The

IT BECAME A POINT OF CIVIC PRIDE TO HAVE A WATER APPROVAL SIGN ON THE OUTSKIRTS OF TOWN.

biggest problem he faced was malfunctioning septic systems. As late as the early 1970s, there were an estimated 1,000 malfunctioning septic tanks in rural Pulaski County and 4,000 surrounding Beaver Lake in North Arkansas. In 1972, after years of political negotiations with the Home Builders Association the legislature passed Act 402 which regulated the construction, installation, operation and maintenance of individual sewage disposal systems. Prior to this Act, the Division of Sanitary Services was receiving about 10,000 complaints a year and there had been a gradual increase in water borne disease. As the Act took effect and the new septic systems were installed the complaints and problems began to decrease. Speaking of Kellogg and his Department in a 1982 interview, Dr. Easley said: "When you turn on the tap to fill your glass you don't give it a second thought as to whether it contains anything harmful."

THE OTHER INFECTIOUS DISEASES

The various infectious diseases that had plagued the state for the last two centuries had been reduced in frequency but they had not gone away. These illnesses taxed the investigative abilities of the public health nurses, the county sanitarians, local physicians and the communicable disease staff of the Board of Health.

Venereal Disease, specifically syphilis and gonorrhea continued to be prevalent. In the mid-1940s penicillin became available for the treatment of both diseases. In 1948, there were 24,400 cases of VD reported and treated in the state of Arkansas. Prenatal screening for syphilis became a routine and in the early 1950s mandatory pre-martial testing was begun. By 1953 programs were in place to focus attention on the contacts of those who were infected and by 1954 the rates of syphilis and gonorrhea had dropped to 1,351 and 1,553, respectively. Dr. Easley attributed the obvious success to a combination of a treatment that created minimal interference with people's lives and rapid follow up of contacts. In the midst of all of the success, the federal funding for public health was slashed. When Dr. Easley was interviewed in 1985 about the reduction in funds in the early 1950s, the sadness in his voice was apparent. Since there was no money for diagnosis, treatment and the follow-up of contacts, the burden fell on the shoulders of the busy private physicians. There is good evidence that less than 13 percent of the VD was being reported by the private medical community and there was almost no contact follow-up. As with polio immunization, funds for the diagnosis and treatment of indigent clients were almost non-existent. Between 1954 and 1959, there was a tripling of the yearly rates of both syphilis and gonorrhea. In the early 1960s, the Board of Health created an intensive program of education involving the physicians, encouraging them to accept the services of the interviewer/investigators that the Board provided. To the extent that this program was successful the numbers did begin to drop and by 1970 some real progress was being made, especially with syphilis.

Tuberculosis, like syphilis, was not going to go away. Streptomycin emerged as a potential cure for TB in the mid-1940s. It was first used on a critically ill patient in 1944 and the results were remarkable; but, there were several major problems—the drug caused intense vertigo and kidney damage making patients hesitant to take it; if that wasn't enough the TB bacteria almost immediately began to develop resistance to it. Within a few years other drugs became available including p-aminosalicylic acid, isoniazid, pyrazinamide, cycloserine, ethambutol, and rifampin. These drugs allowed the physicians to develop multi-drug regimens that could overcome the problems of resistance.

Even with an adequate number of beds the sanatoriums had developed other problems. A large number of patients simply refused to stay. In 1953 there were over 10,000 known TB patients in the state of Arkansas. At least 1,100 of those patients were actively infectious and living at home against medical advice. In 1951, Dr. Herron commented in his report to the Arkansas Medical Society that: "It is interesting to note that almost half of the patients dying of TB die in their home. Since these terminal cases are highly contagious, a grave potential spread of the disease is thus produced. One appalling thing is that ten percent or 200 of the new cases reported during the year were first reported by death certificate."

In the 1940s, four mobile X-ray units and four stationary units were actively doing broad surveys attempting to identify asymptomatic cases of TB.

By the mid-1950s the decision was made to eliminate the mass X-ray screening in the low risk parts of the state and focus the attention where most of the disease occurred. In 1958 Chest Clinics in three separate communities were developed in an attempt to deal with TB on a local basis. By 1960 there were 12 of these clinics operating with private physicians trained by the Board of Health in TB evaluation.

In addition to the new clinics, TB skin testing had been introduced and the confidence level in its accuracy was beginning to rise. Soon public health nurses in 22 counties were doing skin testing.

Hermione Swindoll is another of those heroines of the public health nursing in Arkansas. She was born in Shiloh, Mississippi, raised in Hazen, Arkansas and graduated from the University of Tennessee School of Nursing in 1941. She served in the Army Nurse Corp during the war and in 1949 became a staff nurse at the Little Rock City Health Department. In the late 1950s she obtained a MPH from Tulane and in 1959 returned to Arkansas as an officer of the U.S. Public Health Service assigned to the State Board of Health as a nurse consultant in TB. Mary Gaither, Director of Connect Care at the Health Department, remembers her as a wonderful, smart, kind, no-nonsense lady who was devoted to her patients and her job. In 1961 Dr. Paul Reagan, a young aggressive physician, became the Director of Tuberculosis Control. Ms. Swindoll and Dr. Reagan were instrumental in moving Arkansas away from sanatorium-based care to community-based treatment and care. One of Reagan's first acts was to dramatically increase the number of Chest Clinics and begin looking for ways to enhance in-community programs. He traveled to the Booneville Sanatorium and then on to McRae; Reagan pronounced the facility at McRae "appalling." Early on he began pushing to have all TB services in the state including the sanatoriums under one roof. He brought in consultants who he knew would agree with his approach. One of his mantras was the "uninterrupted medical care of the individual from first suspicion through diagnosis, medical management at home or in a hospital, and ultimate rehabilitation."

In 1968, Reagan and Swindoll began a pilot project at Jefferson Memorial Hospital in Pine Bluff to provide short term hospital care for acutely ill TB patients. In the first year, 209 patients were admitted, 87 were new treatment cases that required only 33 days of in-hospital care. This was in contrast to the Sanatorium where in the first six months of 1967, 96 patients were admitted to the sanatorium and 33 left against medical advice. The new program of short term hospitalization with 18 months of out-patient therapy had a 95 percent success.

Dr. Reagan left the state in 1968 and for several years, Ms. Swindoll with the assistance of Dr. Joseph H. Bates at the Veterans Hospital, managed TB care for the state. In 1972 Dr. Bates convinced Dr. William Stead, an international expert in TB, to join him at the VA in Little Rock and in 1974 Dr. Stead moved to the Arkansas Department of Health and successfully managed the TB control program until his retirement in 1998. Ms. Swindoll ran the day-to-day workings of the program until her retirement in 1979.

McRae was ordered closed in 1966 because of desegregation and declining population. In 1971, as part of a re-organization of state government, the Board of Health officially became the Department of Health. As a part of that reshuffling the Sanatorium at Booneville was made part of the Department of Health. On February 26, 1973, the last seven patients were discharged and the TB facility was closed.

Dr. Joseph H. Bates, Chief Science Officer at the Arkansas Department of Health, points proudly to the fact that we have had almost no resistant TB because of work of Swindoll, Reagan and Stead and their program of treatment and consistent follow-up through the Chest Clinics of the Health Department.

It would be wonderful if this were the end of the story with TB but like syphilis, TB has continued to be a tough and persistent problem.

Typhoid fever is another of those ancient diseases that persisted into mid-20th century Arkansas. The illness is caused by the bacterium, Salmonella typhi. In early Arkansas history it was one of those diseases that fell under the category of Remittent or Recurring fevers. It is most often transmitted by the ingestion of food or water contaminated with fecal material of an infected person. The illness often begins with fever, headache, malaise and a very slow heart rate. After a week the patient begins to experience marked confusion with red spots on the chest and abdomen. Soon abdominal pain and diarrhea with frequent stools begins. In the worst cases, the patient develops gastrointestinal bleeding followed by dehydration. In the 20th century, death from typhoid was uncommon but about five percent of those who were infected with typhoid became asymptomatic carriers of the bacteria.

The advent of chlorinated water and adequate sewer systems lead to a dramatic reduction in the transmission of typhoid fever by mid-century and most mini-epidemics of typhoid could be traced to one of these asymptomatic carriers. The infamous Mary Mallon, "Typhoid Mary," a New York cook who was infected with the bacterium is the classic example. By early in the 1960s, almost all of the typhoid in Arkansas could be traced to one of 130 carriers scattered throughout the state. The carriers were identified by local public health nurses doing excellent investigative work. When a carrier was

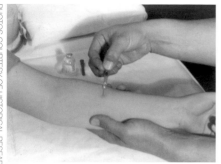

TB SKIN TESTING HAD BEEN INTRODUCED AND THE CONFIDENCE LEVEL IN ITS ACCURACY WAS BEGINNING TO RISE. SOON PUBLIC HEALTH NURSES IN 22 COUNTIES WERE DOING SKIN TESTING.

positively identified by doing stool cultures they were asked to sign an agreement stating they would not work as a food handler. In a number of rural cases, the carrier had cows and sold their un-pasteurized milk, part of the agreement was that they would cease and desist from this activity as well. Slowly with careful investigative workup, follow up and improved water systems, typhoid began to diminish in frequency in the state.

Two other closely related bacterial gastrointestinal illnesses, Salmonellosis and Shigellosis, were common in the early 1960s. A high percentage of the cases were found in northeast Arkansas specifically—Craighead, Mississippi, Crittenden and Poinsett counties.

In addition to the bacterial gastrointestinal illness, there were a number of viral gastrointestinal mini-epidemics that popped up around the state during the 1950s and 1960s. Since polio is primarily a gastrointestinal virus it was no great surprise that the other viruses such as the ECHO and Coxsackie viruses showed themselves during outbreaks of polio. In 1951 viral hepatitis became a reportable disease. Nationwide and in Arkansas, the years 1961 and 1965 saw high rates of hepatitis focused mainly among school children and young adults. It would be another decade before it would be easy to clearly identify the differences between viral and serum hepatitis. The intestinal parasites hookworm, roundworm and ameba were routinely reported from all around the state.

Two other traditional childhood diseases still occurred in sufficient numbers to be of concern.

Diphtheria is a severe sore throat with high fever, extremely large lymph nodes in the neck that can often significantly interfere breathing effort. The D of the DPT immunization is diphtheria toxoid. Like tetanus this is a completely preventable disease. With increasing immunization the reservoir of disease diminished.

Whooping Cough, or pertussis, is another of those diseases that was slowing disappearing. The P of the DPT immunization is pertussis. The classic symptoms of pertussis are intense bouts of coughing with inspiratory "whooping" followed by vomiting. The illness was most serious in children less than one year of age. As late as 1943, there were 93 deaths in Arkansas from whooping cough but by 1962 that number had dropped to three.

One interesting note about the development of the vaccine for pertussis relates to Dr. Margaret Pittman. Pittman was born in 1901 near Prairie Grove in northwest Arkansas. Her father was a country doctor and as a child, she and her sister helped with administering smallpox vaccine in her father's office. She was a bright young lady and in 1923 graduated from Hendrix. She earned a master's degree and Ph.D. in bacteriology from the University of Chicago. In 1936 she joined the National Institute of Health, where, for most of her career, she was involved in the testing and standardization of vaccines. She was most noted for her work on pertussis vaccine.

During the Depression, large parts of the wildlife population of the state were killed off and it was not until the late 1940s and the emergence of an active Game and Fish Commission that the wildlife populations began to rebound: chief among these were white-tail deer, turkey, raccoon and rabbits.

Tularemia is commonly called "rabbit fever" and can occur when a hunter with a cut or sore on his hand cleans a rabbit. The bacteria, Francisella tularensis, enters through the open sore and soon the patient is running fever and has large inflamed lymph nodes usually in the arm and axillary area. In 1964, there were 60 reported cases in 27 counties. Early on, Streptomycin and tetracycline were found to be effective in the treatment of this malady. Dr. Roger Bost, a prominent Arkansas pediatrician, was the first to report that streptomycin was effective in the treatment of tularemia in 1946.

Leptospirosis is an illness caused by bacteria, Leptospria, and the individual is infected through contact with the urine of an infected animal or the exposed flesh of the animal. It is rather uncommon in humans and as such is often misdiagnosed. In the worst cases it may cause high fever and even meningitis like symptoms. It is not usually fatal but can be severe in cases, with relapses of illness.

As the wild animal population increased there was an upsurge in the number of animal bites in humans. In the first half of 1959, there were 468 bites reported to the Board of Health. The majority of these were in children. In that same timeframe, 130 cases of rabies were reported in animals. One half were in foxes and about a third in dogs. Rabies is a viral illness and if the animal proved to be rabid, a 14 dose round of vaccination was advised.

Rocky Mountain Spotted Fever, a rickettsial infection, which is transmitted with the bite of an infected tick, occurs primarily during the spring and summer. It usually manifests by high fever and a measles-like rash that starts at the wrist and spread to the rest of the body. In the 1950s, the newly available tetracycline products were found somewhat effective treating the illness.

Though technically not from a wild animal, the illness Brucellosis is caused by the bacteria, Brucella. It is a common cause of abortion in cattle and can be transmitted to humans when there is contact with the placenta or other tissue products. It can also be transmitted in milk infected with the bacteria. In 1963

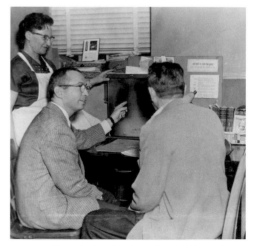

DR. PAUL REAGAN WAS AN INTENSE CRUASADER AGAINST TUBERCULOSIS. HE WAS INSTRUMNETAL IN DEVELOPING THE CHEST CLINIC PROGRAM OF TB CONTROL IN ARKANSAS.

there were 10 cases reported in the state, the majority were young males who had assisted in the birthing of a calf or a spontaneous abortion.

The Viral encephalitis problems identified in Arkansas during this time were Eastern Equine encephalitis, Western Equine encephalitis and St. Louis encephalitis. In horses the illness presented as a sleeping sickness and was often fatal. It was thought that birds were the natural host and various mosquitos acted as the vector. Eastern Equine can be fatal depending of the adequacy of supportive care. In 1962, there were a large number of cases in horses but only seven in humans.

Histoplasmosis is a fungal lung disease that was once thought to be rare in Arkansas. With the advent of readily available chest x-rays and skin tests for both TB and Histoplasmosis, it became clear that it was common and that 98 percent of those who live in the Mississippi River system had been exposed and had positive skin tests.

Blastomycosis, a fungus, was known to be endemic to Arkansas but its importance as a source of disease had not been established. There had been 102 confirmed cases in the preceding 40 years and was widely distributed across the state. It was apparent that dogs also suffered from this illness. Part of the problem with Blastomycosis was that it mimics so many other chronic diseases such as TB and a variety of skin diseases

Tetanus is caused by the toxin of the bacteria, Clostridia tetani. In a full blown case, every muscle in the body is in spasm and nothing relieves it. (A brief note from the author, I was a resident at Baptist Medical Center in Little Rock in 1973 and participated in the care of a man from Patterson on the Cache River. We watched him die and there was nothing we could do about it.) The first inactive tetanus toxoid vaccine went into production in 1924. It was successful in dramatically reducing the incidence of tetanus during World War II. As late as the early 1960s, there were still 10 to 15 cases a year, most in east Arkansas. It was and is a preventable disease.

DENTISTRY AND PUBLIC HEALTH

Arkansas dentistry has a long history going back to the earliest days of the territory. Early dentistry in Arkansas was primarily performed by physicians or itinerant dentists who moved from one small town to the next. As with physicians, most of the early dentists did a preceptorship with an established dentist for several years and then put out their own shingle. By the 1880s, university-trained dentists were beginning to take the upper hand and in 1887 the Arkansas Dental Association was formed. In 1915 the first dental examiners were established for the purpose of licensure. The first real foray into the public's health was an article published in 1900 by a Dr. Gillespie of the Arkansas Dental Association called "Dental Education for the Masses." In 1911 Dr. J.W. Barnett, J.D. Jordon, T.M. Milan and Edgar Smith instituted a short-lived program of dental care for the school children of the Little Rock school system.

By 1928, dentists in Texarkana, with the assistance of the Junior Service League, did dental surveys and provided care in the school system of their city. During this same time Little Rock dentists with the financial support of the Arkansas Federation of Women's Clubs examined and provided dental care for 3,072 low income children in Little Rock schools. The year 1930 saw a nationwide effort to promote dental care; the Arkansas project was headed up by Dr. F.D. Woods of Little Rock

In July 1938, the State Dental Association appointed a Dental Advisory Committee who met with the State Health Officer, the director of the division of Maternal and Child health and a dental consultant for the U.S. Public Health Service. Seventeen part-time dentists were added to county health departments across the state. What small amount of money that was available for dental services came through the Children's Bureau and Title VI funds from the U.S. Public Health Service. In 1939 and 1940, two dentists were hired and traveled the state with trailers equipped as dental offices providing limited services through local health units.

After the first two years of cooperation but very little money, the Dental Health Association pushed for the first full-time dental health director in the Board of Health. Dr. R. P. Spurlin Jr. who practiced in Berryville and had done public health work in Kentucky was named to the directorship. For the first 13 years of the dental program, it was a subdivision of the Maternal and Child Health.

In 1901, Dr. Fredrick McKay, a dentist in Colorado Springs, Colorado, had noticed that many of his patients had mottled teeth; the locals called it Colorado brown stain. Despite the staining, these patients had few cavities. In 1909, Dr. F.L. Robertson of Bauxite, Arkansas noticed a similar condition after a deep well was dug for the town. The town of Bauxite sat on top of the largest deposit of bauxite in the continental U. S. and a chemist who worked for Aluminum Company of America determined that the source of the mottled teeth was the water that contained 13.7 parts per million of fluoride. Over a decade, researchers worked to find safe levels of fluoride that protected teeth from decay but did not cause the staining. In 1935, the U.S. Public Health Service convinced the city of Grand Rapids, Michigan to add fluoride to their water supply. Between 1935 and 1950 the project demonstrated a 60 percent reduction in tooth decay.

During the late 1940s, the U.S. Public Health Service performed a number of fluoridation application demonstration projects in Arkansas. In 1950, West Helena became the first city in Arkansas to fluoridate their water. During the 1950s, increasing numbers of communities in Arkansas chose to add fluoride to their water. In 1958, after six years of fluoridation in the cities of Springdale and Jonesboro, both cities showed a 50 to 60 percent reduction in cavities. Increasingly, communities followed their lead. By the turn of the 21st century, 65 percent of the population in Arkansas was served by fluoridation.

On July 26, 1951, the Arkansas Board of Health adopted a resolution endorsing and recommending fluoridation of drinking water supplies. Dr. Glen Kellogg was one of the big proponents of fluoridation. In 1950, Dr. Don Hamm of Clarksville was appointed by Governor Sid McMath as the first dentist to be a member of the Board of Health. In 1953, Dr. H. Shirley Dwyer was appointed director of Dental Hygiene with the Board of Health and Miss Frances Goodenough, a dental hygienist, was provided by the U.S. Public Health Service for dental health activities, education and research. In 1954, the State Board of Health created the Division of Dental Health.

MATERNAL AND INFANT CARE

Among the most important pillars of the public's health is maternal, infant and child care. Since 1912 and the establishment of the Federal Children's Bureau, the Sheppard-Towner Act of 1921 and the Crippled Children's Fund in 1936, the governmental bodies of this country have acknowledged the importance of this area to the health of the country. Hand and hand with this recognition has been the progress of childhood education. After the end of World War II, both areas took dramatic steps forward, often together.

Once significant progress was made in dealing with the midwife problems and the infant and maternal mortality began to fall, public health began to turn its attention to a series of other important issues.

Statewide public health programs of vision and hearing testing in the schools were implemented in conjunction with the State Department of Education.

Nutritional consultants were hired and the Board of Health revised the Arkansas Diet Manual, making it available to doctors, hospitals and schools.

Statistical data demonstrated that accidents were far and away the most common cause of death among children age one to 19 years with motor vehicle accidents, drowning and poisoning leading the way. In 1958, the first poison control center was established in Little Rock and by 1965 there were poison control centers established in Osceola, Harrison, Fort Smith, El Dorado and Pine Bluff.

In 1955, with strong lobbying from Governor Orval Faubus, the Arkansas Legislature passed Act 6 creating the Arkansas Children's Colony in Conway, the first facility to serve developmentally disabled children in Arkansas. Funding for the building of the home and operating expenses came from a variety of sources. Several organizations acted as ongoing sponsors including the Kiwanis Clubs of Arkansas and the Arkansas Federation of Women's Clubs. Early on, the colony housed 256 residents but by the early 1970s it had grown to accommodate more than a 1,000.

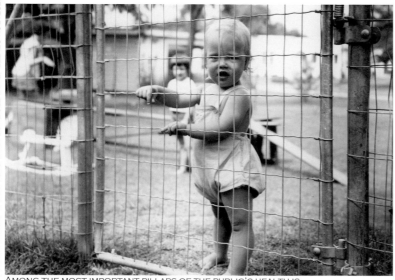

AMONG THE MOST IMPORTANT PILLARS OF THE PUBLIC'S HEALTH IS MATERNAL, INFANT AND CHILD CARE.

In 1956, the Board of Health received a grant from the federal government to set up a diagnostic center for the evaluation of mentally challenged children. Although it began as a strictly diagnostic service that worked with the Children's Colony and the Child Guidance Center at the medical school, it soon evolved into setting up in-home programs for many of these children. By the early 1970s, the program was renamed the Handicapped Child Center.

In the late 1940s, there were few trained obstetricians or pediatricians in the state of Arkansas. Almost all deliveries were performed by family doctors and black midwives. In 1945, Dr. Eva Dodge began her career at the University of Arkansas Medical School. She became acting head of the Department of Obstetrics in 1946. A devotee of Margaret Sanger, founder of Planned Parenthood, Dr. Dodge was an outspoken advocate of family planning and soon had junior and senior medical students participating in rural public health maternity clinics. Part of the logic behind the medical students working in these rural clinics was for their own experience but additionally it was used to assist the midwife training program to identify and funnel complicated at-risk patients to the University. At that point Dr. Dodge was working closely with the Board of Health and Dr. Rothert and Dr. Vida Gordon at the Crippled Children's program. In June 1949, these three ladies were instrumental in convincing the Crippled Children's Program to initiate a grant for $35,000 to establish a department of pediatrics at the medical school.

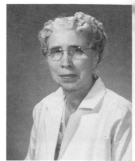

IN 1946, DR. EVA DODGE BECAME ACTING HEAD OF THE DEPARTMENT OF OBSTETRICS.

A fledgling public health in-home care program for premature newborns had begun in 1944 and with the pushing of Dr. Rothert and Dr. Dodge it continued to gain steam. Most neonatal deaths are associated with prematurity, congenital malformation and low-birth weight. Good prenatal care, nutritional counseling and follow-up after the birth had been shown to be effective in reducing the neonatal deaths. By 1953, public health nurses made 45,000 home and office visits to mothers, infants and children. By 1955, 50 percent of public health nurse visits were for maternal and child health. By the late 1950s fewer and fewer deliveries were done by midwives and the neonatal and maternal deaths rates were dropping. In 1959 a trial program to check for phenylketonuria in newborns was begun; demonstrations had shown that a diet low in phenylalanine in those patients was effective in preventing a form of mental retardation if started early enough.

In 1961, the Jefferson County Special Project for Premature Infants was begun. It was a program funded primarily by the federal government through Crippled Children and involved comprehensive prenatal care with close supervision and in-home care of the infants with portable incubators and frequent nurse visits after delivery. It became clear early in the project that a holistic approach was what was needed; soon, they were providing a variety of services. As a part of the maturity evaluation, Pap smears were performed and once the pregnancy was complete, family planning and birth control were instituted. Almost all of the women and children were well below the poverty line, but those who were running the program did not attempt to enforce means testing; if someone asked for care they got it. Dr. Dodge had worked closely with the early development and testing of intrauterine devices (IUD) as a birth control device and early in the program they used a large number of IUDs. When birth control pills came on the market, the program negotiated a reduced price for the pills and began switching to oral contraceptives. The Maternal and Infant Care project covered the children up through age two. By the late 1960s, a Child and Youth Program began and covered the children up through school age. By this time Medicaid services were available and beginning to provide financing for some of the further care.

In 1964, Dr. Rex Ramsey became head of the Child and Maternal Division at the Board of Health. When interviewed in the early 1990s it is easy to hear in his comments that he was especially proud of the Pine Bluff project and all of the good it did.

Another important project of the late 1960s was the passage of Act 244 of 1967. The Vaccination Assistance Act of 1962 provided the money for the Sabin Polio mass inoculations. In addition funds were made available for the purchase of vaccines for preschoolers and for the development of a more comprehensive and effective delivery of immunization services. As late as 1964 surveys revealed that immunization protection was still low for all age groups. In 1967, at the insistence and prodding of the Board of Health, the Arkansas Legislature enacted mandatory immunization requirements for kindergarten through twelve grades. Over the years, as the various immunizations have changed, the law has been updated twice in 1973 and again in 1997.

HEALTH INSURANCE

Prior to 1920 medical care costs were low and the truth was there was little that health professionals could do. Most care was provided in the home. The 1920s and 1930s saw a significant increase in technology such as X-ray and the beginnings of the development of the modern hospital. Even at that, the cost of illness was primarily the cost of lost wages. Health insurance in that time was more what we would think of as disability insurance.

In 1920, Dr. Fred Jones, a black physician and entrepreneur in Little Rock, offered a hospital plan designed to offset future hospital visits for two black fraternal organizations. In 1923, a group of white physicians joined together to create Trinity Hospital in Little Rock and in 1931 the hospital began a pre-payment program where an individual could receive all of his care for $2.00 a month or $2.50 for the a family group. To the Pulaski County Medical Society and Arkansas Medical Society, this smacked of socialism and state medicine; for the next 15 years, the physicians and their hospital were censured and removed from the roles of the county and state medical society.

It seems that the medical society was once again fighting a losing battle because by 1945 there were four other prepayment programs in Arkansas: a paper mill in Camden, one in Dierks and two consumer-sponsored groups— one in Fort Smith and the other in Prescott.

In 1929, a group of Dallas school teachers contracted with Baylor University to provide 21 days of hospital coverage a year for $6.00.

The American Hospital Association eventually embraced this type program and called it Blue Cross. As prepaid hospital plans became more popular, the American Medical Association got into the act and created a plan to cover physician's services adopting the name Blue Shield.

After several decades of fighting any type of health insurance, the Arkansas Hospital Association and the Arkansas Medical Society joined forces with the Arkansas Farm Bureau and in 1948 formed Arkansas Blue Cross and Blue Shield; it was just in time. In 1940, 20 million were covered by health insurance in the U. S. and in 1950 that number had grown to 60 million.

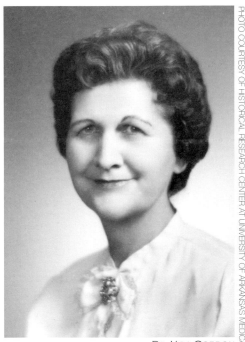

DR. VIDA GORDON

In the late 1930s, an attempt was made to create national health insurance as a part of the initial Social Security Act. Intense lobbying on the part of the AMA prevented its inclusion. In 1949, one year after the Arkansas insurance group formed, the AMA and Arkansas Medical Society lobbied and helped to ensure the defeat of a proposal for comprehensive national health insurance by Congress and President Truman. Every physician who was a member of the organizations was charged a $25 fee for their lobbying efforts.

In the 1950s, commercial insurance got into the act and by 1958 over half of Americans had some form of health insurance. During the Eisenhower Administration, very little was done but with the election of John F. Kennedy in 1960 and especially when the Democrats won a majority in Congress in 1964 the stage was set for the passage of Medicare and Medicaid in 1965.

Medicare provided health insurance, to people age 65 and older, regardless of income or medical history. Eighty percent of adults over 60 were at or near the poverty line; if they had health insurance they paid three times as much for the same coverage. The passage of Medicare also advanced the cause of desegregation by mandating common facilities.

Medicaid was created as a means-tested companion program designed to provide coverage for low-income families, low income pregnant women and the disabled.

As with earlier initiatives, these bills were fought tooth and nail by the medical profession and conservative politicians.

Just as with the Social Security programs of the 1930s, Medicare and Medicaid altered the course of the public's health in a dramatic fashion.

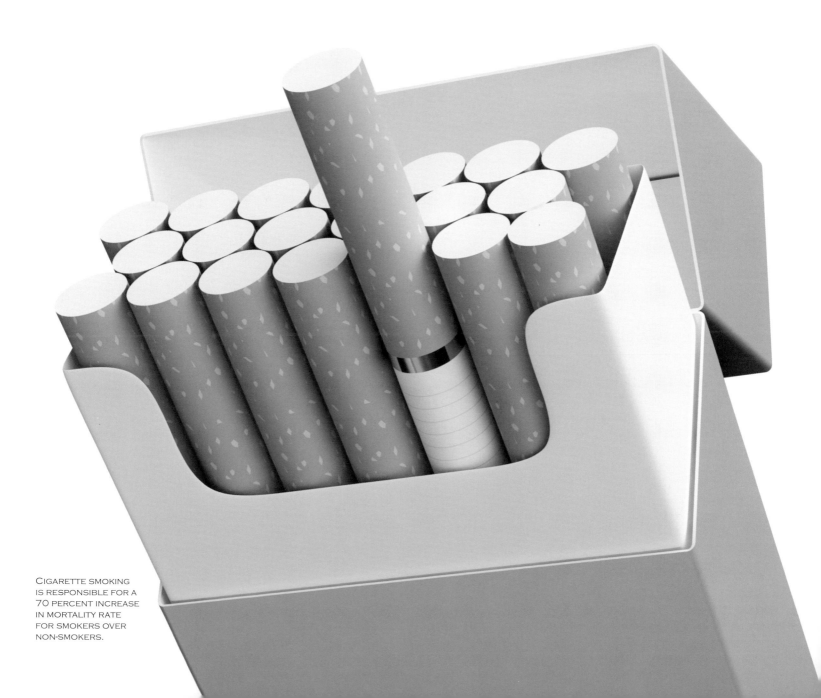

CIGARETTE SMOKING IS RESPONSIBLE FOR A 70 PERCENT INCREASE IN MORTALITY RATE FOR SMOKERS OVER NON-SMOKERS.

CHAPTER EIGHT
A CHANGE OF PRIORITIES

The 1970s were a time of great change in the public's health of Arkansas and the nation. Desegregation was now the law of the land; that and the passage of Medicare and Medicaid in the mid-1960s provided increasing access to health care for those who had none. The country was mired in an unpopular war. The Voting Rights Act of 1965 enfranchised African-American voters and they in turn helped to elect Winthrop Rockefeller as the first Republican governor in 100 years; despite good intentions he was unable to work with the legislature. He was followed by Dale Bumpers, David Pryor and Bill Clinton; three progressive racially-moderate governors who were intent on improving the quality of life in Arkansas for the average citizen. In the 1950s and 1960s, Arkansas lost population and, for the eastern third of the state, this continued for the rest of the 20th century. Along with the loss of population the health care providers in rural parts of the state were aging and there was no one to replace them; hospitals and clinics were closing in all of the rural areas. King Cotton had been replaced by soybeans, rice, corn and poultry. The economic power base had shifted from the Delta to Central and Northwest Arkansas. The U.S. Space Program dramatically increased our engineering and research capacity and with it came an explosion of new medical technologies and medicines. In 1963, the birth control pill created an unobtrusive mechanism for family planning and unwanted pregnancy; as with any new technology, birth control pills and penicillin turned out to be a pair of double-edged swords, the sexual revolution they engendered resulted in an increase in the numbers of sexual partners, sexual encounters and subsequently increased STDs.

The public health services of Arkansas were going through a significant transition. When the Board of Health was created in 1913, the offices and labs were housed on the second floor of the Old State House in downtown Little Rock. They shared space with the newly formed medical school, in fact, the Board of Health lab doubled as the lab for the school. Linnie Beauchamp, the first nurse supervisor for the Board of Health, related that her office was the cloak room for the old Senate chambers. The building was in terrible shape and several women's groups were interested in removing the tenants and doing major renovations to the building. In 1923 they got their wish when the legislature provided $17,000 to renovate a portion of the basement of the new State Capitol. When interviewed in 1985, Dr. Easley commented that when he came to work in the late 1930s the space was small and cramped and the lab was in a portion of the basement that still had dirt floors. By 1942, the state and federal government worked together and built a Health Department building on the west end of the Capitol Mall. Because of a proliferation of bureaus and divisions that building was too small when they moved in. In the mid-1960s, Governor Faubus with coaxing from Dr. J.T. Herron agreed to add his backing to the building of a new health department building and, in 1969, Governor Rockefeller dedicated the new modern facility on West Markham. As with the building in 1942, additions were needed almost immediately and a south wing of the building was added. In 2006, the mandated services for the lab had grown and a new lab building was added to the complex.

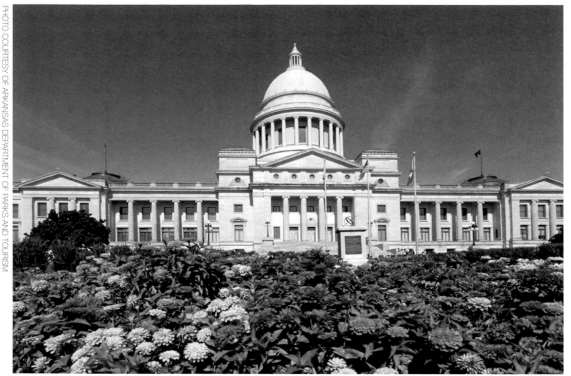

IN THE MID-1920S, THE ARKANSAS BOARD OF HEALTH MOVED FROM THE OLD STATE HOUSE TO THE BASEMENT OF THE NEW CAPITOL BUILDING.

In addition to new quarters the Board of Health officially acquired a new name in 1971. Newly-elected Governor Dale Bumpers forced through a re-organization of state government collapsing 60 state agencies into 13 cabinet level departments; the Arkansas Health Department was the result of this change. The Board of Health continued as an advisory board but the director of the Health Department was now a member of the governor's cabinet.

With the new status Dr. Herron sent a request to the governor for an increase in the budget and a substantial raise for the director. He noted in his request that there were at least four people in the department with less seniority, less responsibility and more pay. The department did receive an increase in the budget but the salary increase was ignored. On December 16, 1971, a dissatisfied Dr. Herron resigned to take a job in Oregon for better pay and less stress. Governor Bumpers named Dr. John Harrell as the new director of the department. Dr. Harrell had been the director of the Arkansas Child Development Center of the Health Department. The salary for the new director was almost twice that of Dr. Herron. Over the next 27, years there would be six different directors for the Department of Health. During Dr. Harrell's tenure some progress was made toward re-organization of the department. He was, however, embroiled in a minor but illegal travel voucher fund that embarrassed the governor. By 1973 he left for a different job in Decatur, Georgia. Harrell was followed by Dr. Rex Ramsey, a long-term pediatrician with the Maternal and Infant program. This was a time of austerity in state government and most of the money came from federal programs. It was during this time that nurse practitioners and physician assistants began to appear in maternal and infant programs for the medically underserved. In 1979, when Bill Clinton became governor, he did not reappoint Dr. Ramsey and instead brought in Dr. Robert Young, a West Virginian and an expert in rural health development. He almost immediately began to ruffle feathers in the state, first among the old time staff of the Health Department. "When I looked at the organization chart it looked more like a disorganization chart," he commented to an *Arkansas Gazette* reporter. One of his first acts was to hire a health planner from California, begin eliminating positions in the Little Rock office and re-distribute those jobs across the state. The next battle was over a grant for rural health that was opposed by the Arkansas Health Systems Agency, a planning body, and the Arkansas Medical Society. It would be this fight that was his downfall and in January 1981 he left for a job in Kentucky. Governor Frank White appointed Dr. Ben Saltzman, a Mountain Home physician and stalwart in the Arkansas Medical Society. Several years earlier he had a heart attack and while he was recuperating Dr. Tom Bruce, Dean of the Medical School, enticed him to come to Little Rock and take over the leadership of the newly-formed Family Practice Residency in an attempt to lure more young doctors into the smaller towns of Arkansas. For several reasons his six years as director of the Health Department were

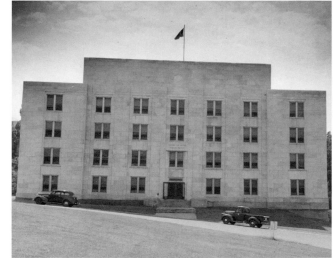

DURING WORLD WAR II THE BOARD OF HEALTH HAD OUTGROWN ITS SPACE IN THE CAPITOL. WITH THE HELP OF THE FEDERAL GOVERNMENT A BUILDING WAS CONSTRUCTED ON THE WEST END OF THE CAPITOL MALL. BY THE TIME THE BUILDING WAS BUILT, IT WAS TOO SMALL.

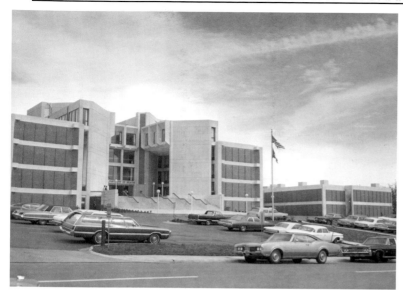

At the urging of Dr. Herron, the new Department of Health was built in the late 1960s.

somewhat tranquil; according to Dr. Davis Fitzhugh, Saltzman acted more as a caretaker. One reason for the tranquility was the lack of money. Most of the money for running the Health Department came from the federal government and the Reagan administration dramatically reduced the funds available for public health. A second reason for the relative quietness of the Department had to do with the fact that Dr. Saltzman did not take a single step that would inflame the Arkansas Medical Society. His replacement was Dr. Jocelyn Elders, an African-American and a pediatric endocrinologist from the University of Arkansas Medical Center. In her biography, Dr. Elders indicated that before she took her post at the Health Department, public health had not been high on her list of ambitions: "In the whole time as a working pediatrician I hadn't ever spent more than five minutes at a stretch thinking about public health." Upon taking the job she quickly immersed herself in the problems that faced the state. As a pediatrician she had been aware of the problems of teen pregnancy. She was always known for being outspoken and as director of the Health Department this was no different. With the backing of her boss, Bill Clinton, she began pushing for school-based health clinics and the teaching of sex education in the schools. One of her oft repeated lines was: "Ignorance is not bliss. We've tried it and it didn't work; now, let's try education." Soon she became a lightning rod for criticism of her boss, Bill Clinton. On several occasions she engaged conservative legislators and the religious right over the role of sex education in the schools and school health clinics. In 1993, Dr. Elders left to become the U.S. Surgeon General during President Clinton's first term. Her replacement was Dr. Sandra Nichols, another African-American female, who had completed a residency in family practice at UAMS. When tapped for the job, Nichols was the Medical Director of the Mid-Delta Health Center in Clarendon. During her tenure, she focused on rural health and prevention. In 1997, she left the

state for another job opportunity, and, in 1998, Dr. Fay Boozman, a physician from Springdale, assumed the role as head of the department.

One of Boozman's most important contributions was a public initiative that dedicated all tobacco settlement money to the health of all Arkansans, especially smoking cessation. A number of other states had used the money for shoring up other parts of government, such as building roads and prisons. Governor Huckabee and Boozman worked hard for two years to make sure that didn't happen in Arkansas. In spring 2005, Boozman was killed in a farm accident, and Dr. Paul Halverson, Dr.P.H. (doctorate of Public Health), the first non-medical doctor to hold the office, became director of the Arkansas Health Department. Halverson had been enticed from his job at the CDC in Atlanta to help set up the School of Public Health at UAMS. For 20 years before coming to Arkansas, he had been involved in organizing health and health-related services at large organizations. He had worked for several years as a consultant for the CDC, helping various states organize more efficient and effective public health care.

Since the early 1950s, successive directors have been faced with the problem of dealing with this massive organization; various ones have described it as a piecework quilt or a large jigsaw puzzle with pieces missing. Since the early 1970s, several directors have attempted to re-organize the organization, each running into one obstacle after another, mostly funding. Halverson came to the job with a wonderful background, and he quickly set about evaluating each division, eliminating redundancy and putting the ship on course. He was quick to say that he received excellent cooperation from health department personnel throughout the state and the two governors he served under, Gov. Huckabee and Beebe. In spring 2013, Halverson left to become the head of a new School of Public Health in Indiana. Dr. Nate Smith was appointed to replace him and, as of this writing, has just taken over as the new director.

While the Arkansas Department of Health changed its name, built new buildings, underwent a number of political crises and changes of leadership, the public's health continued unabated.

In early 1967, the federal government passed the Wholesome Meat Act which required that all states have an inspection program for intrastate consumption of meat equal to that of the federal government program for interstate consumption. It came to the attention of the Board of Health that there was a significant gap in the food inspection process in Arkansas. Dr. Herron visited all of the known facilities, took photos and began lobbying the legislature to fund and support a quality meat inspection program. The legislature was convinced. In October 1967, Act 320 created and funded a meat inspection program staffed with five full-time veterinarians, 38 on-site inspectors and 18 part-time private veterinarians who consulted on an as-needed basis. By 1970 the program was certified by the USDA as "equivalent to a Federal inspection" and in May 1971 Dr. Herron signed a formal agreement integrating the state and federal enforcement efforts. Arkansas would be one of 30 states in the U. S. that had a separate state inspection agency. For 10 years the agency was exceedingly busy with more and more inspections required. In 1980, the Arkansas Health Department, like all other phases of state government, went through a major financial crisis;

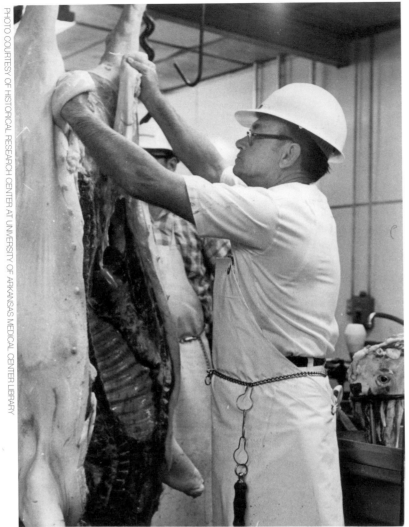

IN MAY 1971, DR. HERRON SIGNED A FORMAL AGREEMENT INTEGRATING THE STATE AND FEDERAL ENFORCEMENT EFFORTS FOR MEAT INSPECTION FOR THE STATE OF ARKANSAS.

meat inspection was hit especially hard with cuts in financing. The following March further major cuts were at hand and sometime during the following year the program was folded into federal management with the USDA.

MENTAL HEALTH

In the middle of the 19th century, Dorothea Dix lobbied the U.S. Congress to create asylums for the mentally ill. When she was unable to convince the national legislature, she began making the rounds of the states. She must have been a very convincing lady because her efforts have been credited with the establishment of 32 hospitals in 18 states. In Arkansas public sentiment for a facility was voiced in the *Arkansas Gazette* as early as the late 1850s. In 1883 the

Arkansas Lunatic Asylum was opened; in 1905 the name was changed to the Arkansas State Hospital for Nervous Diseases, and in 1933 to the Arkansas State Hospital. By 1936 the old facility was full to overflowing and the Benton Farm Colony was opened. It was built large enough to hold 2,000 patients.

In the 1950s and 1960s, Dr. George Jackson was the head of the State Hospital and a close friend of Orval Faubus. In 1960, Dr. Jackson convinced Governor Faubus to build a new facility to replace the old buildings.

By the early 1950s, there were 500,000 individuals in state institutions across the United States. As with tuberculosis sanatoriums there were several changes afoot in the mental health world. In 1942 after a major fire where 492 people died, Dr. Erich Lindeman, a psychiatrist in Boston, opened the first community mental health center to deal with the acute grief reactions of the survivors of the fire. In the early 1950s, chlorpromazine (Thorazine) became available and had a significant impact on the patient populations who were housed in the asylums. Photographic newspaper exposés revealed the desperate lives of those who lived in these facilities.

In 1955, Congress commissioned the Mental Health Study Act and in 1961 they returned with a scathing indictment of the mental health hospitals across the U.S. They made several recommendations; among them were the immediate provision of full-time clinics for the mentally ill in all communities and community-based aftercare and rehabilitation for those leaving mental hospitals.

President Kennedy proposed and Congress passed the Mental Retardation and Community Mental Health Construction Act of 1963. Congress agreed to pass the act but refused to fund the staffing. In 1965 President Johnson amended the act to include staffing for the centers. Almost immediately catchment areas of 75,000-200,000 population began applying for grants to build community mental health centers. In Arkansas, under the leadership of Dr. George Jackson, 12 centers were built around the state.

Between 1955 and 1980 the population of state asylums across the country dropped from 558,000 to 140,000. Many of the patients who were de-institutionalized were simply not ready to be thrown back into the world and the community mental health centers were not equipped with the facilities or manpower to care for them. By the 1980s, the National Mental Health Systems Act was passed. It was an attempt to re-invigorate the community Mental Health Centers and re-direct them to the care of the seriously mentally ill. Less than a year later, Reagan's Omnibus Budget Reconciliation Act of 1981 repealed the Mental Health Systems Act, eliminated all mental health initiatives and all 10 regional federal offices of the National Institutes for Mental Health. Just as would be done with most of the Maternal and Infant monies, all of the money for mental health arrived at the states in the form of block grants. Community Mental Health Centers ultimately made the shift away from the block grant money and to Medicaid.

For the last 30 years, the community mental health system has worked at developing program services for the seriously mentally ill such as Birch Tree Communities, the Gain Program and Stride House that aim to provide a full package of services for the seriously mentally ill in a less restrictive but supportive environment.

IMMUNIZATION AND CHILDCARE

The year of 1971 was a red letter day for all school-aged children and public health officials in the United States. The Surgeon General of the United States Public Health Service issued a ruling that routine primary smallpox vaccination for American children should be discontinued. The scourge that had plagued mankind for seven millennia was no longer a threat in the United States.

Other immunization news in Arkansas was not as good. Despite the efforts of the Health Department and Education Department, less that 50 percent of Arkansas children had completed all of their immunizations by the time they started school. Governor Dale Bumpers and his wife, Betty, had a lifelong interest in childhood education and health. She was a teacher in the Charleston schools and he was the lawyer for the school board when the school was confronted with desegregation. They were instrumental in making Charleston, Arkansas one of the first school districts in the South to peacefully integrate. After her husband became governor of Arkansas, Mrs. Bumpers began working with the health department on an effective childhood immunization program to assure that all children had their immunizations by the time they started school. In 1973, she began a campaign, Every Child by '74, coordinated by Nell Balkman of the Arkansas League of Nursing that later served as a model for immunization programs throughout the rest of the country. Using the power of her husband's office, she commandeered the National Guard, the Agricultural Extension Service, home economists, and all of the volunteer women groups who had made their presence known in the state for the last century. The program was launched in 1973 and was quite successful, immunizing 100,000 children and raising the full immunization rates from near 50 percent to greater than 90 percent. In 1974 Dale Bumpers became the junior senator from Arkansas in Washington. In Washington Betty Bumpers teamed up with President Carter's wife, Rosalynn, and the two ladies created a program called Every Child by Two. The two ladies worked together to implement immunization programs state-by-state. They lobbied for and were instrumental in getting state laws passed in every state making school-entry immunization mandatory. As of 2007, 77 percent of school age children in the United States met all of the vaccination goals and 90 percent met all goals except for the DTap vaccine.

In February 1986, after a Razorback basketball game in Fayetteville, an outbreak of measles began among the student body of the University. It spread rapidly to regional high schools and soon there were 273 cases confirmed in 14 counties. Many of these young people had been immunized for measles prior to 1968. According to Dr. Fitzhugh those early vaccines tended to cause reactions and therefore were often given with gamma globulin. It appears that this and the early timing of the shots interfered with the children's ability to create an immune response to the injection. In response to the mini-epidemic, 92,000 immunizations were given aimed especially at the high schools and college kids of the state and the epidemic was stopped.

The goal of public health's involvement in maternal and infant care is to reduce the numbers of unwanted pregnancies especially in teenagers, to improve the prenatal care of the underserved population and reduce the number of low-birth weight babies. From 1960 to 1980, there was a major drop in infant mortality rates in both white and African-American babies. As noted in an earlier chapter, the Maternal and Infant Care Project and the Children and Youth Project began in the 1960s and during the 1970s began to have a real impact. Most of the care provided was focused on comprehensive care to a large population of underserved women, newborns and children. During the first half of the decade, 25,000 Pap smears a year were done as part of the family planning and prenatal care. In May 1975, an even more aggressive cervical cancer screening campaign was begun. The first year of the program 43,024 women were screened with Pap smears. It was during this timeframe that locally trained nurse practitioners

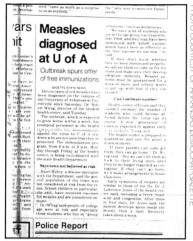

WHEN IT BECAME APPARENT THAT THERE WAS AN EPIDEMIC AT THE UNIVERSITY OF ARKANSAS AT FAYETTEVILLE AND THE SURROUNDING HIGH SCHOOLS, THE DEPARTMENT OF HEALTH SPRANG INTO ACTION AND GAVE 92,000 IMMUNIZATIONS IN A SHORT PERIOD OF TIME.

became quite active in the state. Dr. Robert Merrill, the head of the UAMS Pediatrics department, and Dr. J.O. Cooper were instrumental in starting the nurse training program. At the beginning of the 1970s one of the pieces of the puzzle that was missing was nutrition. In 1967, a National Nutrition Survey revealed dramatic malnutrition among low-income Americans. In 1972, Senators Hubert Humphrey and Robert Dole drafted a program to provided nutrition for Women, Infants and Children (WIC). The Arkansas program began in 1974 with 3,991 clients and by 1984 had grown to 34,000. All of the data available demonstrates that a well-nourished mother gives birth to a healthier baby. In 1976, the Mississippi County Obstetric Nurse Project began because of a lack of obstetric services in that area and by 1977 they were delivering 230 babies per year. In two years, the infant mortality rate in the population serviced dropped dramatically. In 1975, the Sudden Infant Death Syndrome (SIDS) program began in an attempt to detect all SIDS deaths, look for trends and educate the population about the problem. In 1979 the Arkansas Regional Prenatal Program, although not a program of the Arkansas Department of Health, developed the Newborn Transport Service to facilitate transport of critical newborns to UAMS. In this timeframe the Intensive Care Nursery Program at UAMS under the leadership of Dr. Alice Beard developed an aggressive unit dealing with these very ill newborns. Genetic screening for PKU (phenylketonuria) and testing for hypothyroidism were developed; undiagnosed, these two problems lead to mental retardation. In the mid-1970s the Early and Periodic Screening Diagnosis and Treatment Program (EPSDTP) for children from birth to 21 was begun and by the late 1970s they were serving over 24,000 children. In 1978, the Maternal, Infant and Child Health program (MICH) began. This program was designed to

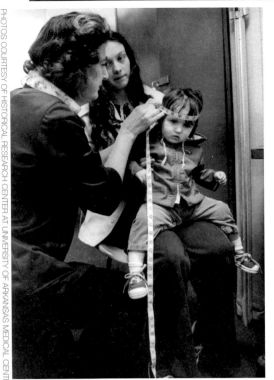

EARLY MATERNAL AND INFANT CARE FOCUSED ON MOTHERS AND INFANTS. IN THE 1970S THEY BEGAN TO EXPAND TO DEAL WITH PROBLEMS OF LATER CHILDHOOD.

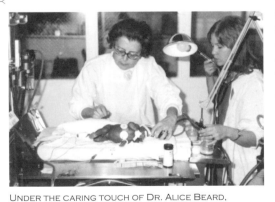

UNDER THE CARING TOUCH OF DR. ALICE BEARD, THE UNIVERSITY OF ARKANSAS MEDICAL SCHOOL DEVELOPED AN AGRESSIVE, INTENSIVE NEWBORN CARE NURSERY DEALING WITH THESE VERY ILL NEWBORNS.

provide comprehensive maternity and pediatric services to all women and children in the state who had little or no means of securing services. There were 10 MICH maternity nurses working under the supervision of a physician, across the state; most were in east and central Arkansas. Once the children were delivered there were eight pediatric nurses who made rounds at all of the local health units.

An important element of all of the programs noted above was family planning. If there was push back to any of these programs it generally had to do with family planning. Each program was adapted to each community. According to Dr. Ramsey and Dr. Fitzhugh, the family planning element was far more successful the farther they got away from the metropolitan areas.

The programs listed above were successful in reducing the rate of low-birth weight and infant mortality. By the early 2000s, 80 percent of women received early prenatal care and 60 of the 75 county health units had prenatal clinical services.

This alphabet soup of initialed programs was funded primarily by federal grants and to some extent Medicaid. In 1980, another of the rounds of austerity struck and most of the financial support for these programs was consolidated into block grants. From that point on about one third of the Maternal and Child Health Grant (MCH) money was spent on prenatal health services in the local health units. Despite the federal cutbacks, the trends were already established. In 1987 Arkansas became one of the first states to take advantage of increased Medicaid eligibility which provided more coverage for children and pregnant women.

One of the best barometers of the health of a nation or a state is the infant mortality rate. Even though the numbers have reduced by as much as 90 percent in the last century, the Arkansas numbers are still above the national average. In 2010 the U.S. averaged 6.4 infant deaths per thousand live births and Arkansas's death rate was 7.3/1,000.

MODERN WASTE

Human activity creates waste. When humans begin to gather in groups, provisions have to be made to deal with that waste. For the first 100 years, public health concerned itself primarily with developing adequate sewer systems and clean water. In the 20th century, the heavy use of petroleum products and manufactured chemicals forced the nation and Arkansas to begin evaluating the long-term effects of these products. No one questioned that DDT almost single-handedly eliminated malaria; the problem with chemicals like DDT was that they didn't go away and their long-term effects were unknown. Waste produced by the human body eventually decomposes but many of these new chemicals become a permanent part of the environment. As early as 1949, the Water Pollution Control Commission was created as a part of the Board of Health. In 1965, the commission was moved out of the Board of Health, the name was changed to Arkansas Pollution Control Commission and air pollution was added to its mandate. In Bumpers' reorganization of 1971, the predecessor to the Arkansas Department of Environmental Quality was created. Since the inception of the department, the director or the chief scientific officer of the Arkansas Health Department has been a member of the board.

In the 1950s, Rachel Carson, a biologist with the U. S. Bureau of Fisheries, began to write about the impact that these chemicals were having on the ocean life. In the early 1960s, she wrote *Silent Spring* detailing the impact of pesticides on human life. Her writing spurred a grassroots movement resulting in a ban on DDT. In 1970, President Richard Nixon signed into law a bill that created the U.S. Environmental Protection Agency.

The Vertac Plant in Jacksonville had originally been part of the Arkansas Ordinance Plant during World War II. The plant was first owned by the Reasor-Hill company in 1948; in the next 30 years, four different companies owned the plant and the last of these was Vertac. All of the companies produced DDT, 2,4,5-T and 2,4-D—a bi-product of 2,4,5-T is dioxin and dioxin had been linked to a number of human diseases such as cancer, disorders of the nervous system and birth defects. Several of the companies buried large numbers of drums containing the production waste of the plant. After complaints from the community, the Arkansas Department of Health and the EPA immediately began investigating. In short order they determined that many of the buried drums were leaking into the soil and ground water around the plant. In conjunction with the Arkansas Health Department, EPA, CDC and the Arkansas Department of Environmental Quality, a team of researchers from Mount Sinai in New York were brought in to perform exams on former Vertac employees, Jacksonville residents and employees of the Jacksonville sewer plant. After some miscommunication, no major human contamination was found, however, fish downstream in Bayou Meto were found to be contaminated. The EPA and the ADEQ sued Vertac and the judge ordered the company to construct a wall around its waste pond. Vertac was forbidden to produce 2,4,5-T and ordered by a federal judge to prevent the spread of dioxin. In 1987 Vertac declared bankruptcy and left behind 29,000 drums of chemicals, about half were above ground, out in the open, and the rest were buried and already leaking.

The EPA declared Vertac a Superfund site and began the process of cleaning up the site. It would take another 12 years and several law suits before all of the dioxin-containing drums were incinerated or moved to a site in Kansas and incinerated, the soil was reclaimed and the buildings destroyed.

In 1986, the U. S. Food and Drug Administration discovered that dairy products produced in Arkansas had been contaminated with heptachlor, another of the pesticides similar to DDT. The chemical is commonly used to kill termites. It seems that a quantity of corn mash contaminated by heptachlor that was supposed to be incinerated as fuel was mistakenly fed to milk cows. This chemical tends to accumulate in breast milk of cows and humans. In a woman who consumes the tainted milk the chemical is then eliminated in her breast milk. The Health Department immediately removed the contaminated milk from the market and had it destroyed. The breast milk of a thousand Arkansas women was tested through the Health Department. The immediate question was: could these women who had consumed the milk product and were breast-feeding continue to breast feed? Early in the controversy, a group of obstetricians from UAMS called a press conference and issued a warning to all breast-feeding mothers to stop immediately. When the testing results were returned there was in fact contamination in most of the breast milk, but it was a very low level and probably no different from the levels that would have been found without the tainted milk.

A month later CDC issued a report that the general population was at no risk and that nursing babies had been at negligible risk. They indicated that the farm families who had handled the feed were at the highest risk primarily because they lived around it and drank the milk from the cows on a daily basis.

THE EMPHASIS OF PUBLIC HEALTH CHANGES— TOBACCO AND CHRONIC DISEASE

"Smoke, smoke, smoke that cigarette
Puff, puff, puff and if you smoke yourself to death
Tell St. Peter at the Golden Gate
That you hates to make him wait
But you just gotta have another cigarette"
Tex Williams, 1947

In the early days of Arkansas, the various intermittent fevers were thought

of as a fact of life; in 1964 tobacco and smoking were just a fact of life and then came the Surgeon General's Report.

At the beginning of the 20th century, most tobacco use was via cigars, pipes or chewed tobacco. A number of advances in the tobacco itself, improved papers and automatic rolling machines made the cigarette cheaper, easier to use and cleaner. At that same time, there was a public health campaign against spitting on the sidewalk because of tuberculosis; the ash tray replaced the cuspidor. Tobacco consumption skyrocketed to the extent that a number of anti-tobacco laws were passed in the early 1920s. Patterned after the anti-alcohol laws, most did not stand the test of time and by the late 1920s all had been repealed except for those related to selling tobacco to children.

In the first half of the 20th century, lung cancer rates began to skyrocket. The American Cancer Society, the National Institute of Health and the Veterans Administration began sponsoring research that would provide conclusive evidence that cigarette smoking was the most important cause of lung cancer and chronic lung disease. The ACS studies also revealed greatly increased illness rates among smokers and a notable shortening of life expectancy of smokers. They established the fact that ex-smokers live longer than smokers, and the longer they went without smoking, the closer their life expectancy approached the life expectancy of those who have never smoked.

By the early 1960s, the evidence against tobacco was overwhelming. The American Cancer Society, the American Heart Association, the National Tuberculosis Association, and the American Public Health Association sent a letter to President Kennedy requesting a national commission on the health hazards of tobacco and smoking. In June 1962, the Surgeon General, Luther L. Terry, announced that he would convene a committee of experts to conduct a comprehensive review of the scientific literature on the smoking question. Terry invited representatives of the four voluntary medical organizations who first proposed the commission, as well as the Food and Drug Administration, the Federal Trade Commission, the American Medical Association and the Tobacco Institute.

On January 11, 1964, The Report of the Surgeon General's Advisory Committee on Smoking and Health was released: Cigarette smoking is responsible for the 70 percent increase in the mortality rate of smokers over non-smokers. Smokers have a 10-fold greater risk of developing lung cancer compared to non-smokers and heavy smokers have at least a 20-fold greater risk. The risk rises with the duration of smoking and diminishes with the cessation of smoking. The report named smoking as the most important cause of chronic lung disease and an important factor in coronary heart disease. It noted that smoking during pregnancy reduced the average weight of newborns.

The battle against smoking was a slow but a progressive process. Each decade has seen progressive drops in the smoking rates. The lung cancer rates began to fall for men in the late 1990s and by 2007 had begun to show a decline in women. As of the latest figures less than 20 percent of the U.S. population continues to use tobacco; the numbers in Arkansas are around the 27 percent range.

At the time the Report was issued in 1964, approximately 51 percent of men

ARKANSAS GAZETTE Monday, March 10, 1986

Major producer recalls 60,000 gallons of milk tainted with pesticide

More recalls possible, state health official says

By Lamar James
GAZETTE STAFF

IN 1986 THE U.S. FOOD AND DRUG ADMINISTRATION DISCOVERED THAT DAIRY PRODUCTS PRODUCED IN ARKANSAS HAD BEEN CONTAMINATED WITH HEPTACHLOR, ANOTHER PESTICIDE SIMILAR TO DDT.

and 33 percent of women smoked. The United States Public Health Service and the American Cancer Society launched an aggressive campaign aimed at informing the public of the dangers of smoking, persuading people to stop, and helping those who were having trouble stopping.

Labeling cigarette packets with the warning: "Caution: Cigarette Smoking May be Hazardous to Your Health" was a start. By January 1971, all TV and radio advertising was eliminated.

In 2006, the Surgeon General issued a finding that there is no risk-free level of exposure to cigarette smoke. Second hand smoke dramatically increases the risk of heart disease and cancer in non-smokers. Children exposed to smoke are at much higher risk of SIDS, respiratory infections and asthma. In April 2006, with strong advocacy by the Arkansas Health Department, Senate Bill 8 was passed that banned smoking in almost all indoor public locations.

As with tobacco, the research that began in earnest after World War II involving heart disease, cancer and stroke began showing dramatic results in the 1960s.

The publication of the early Framingham papers and other major studies began to unfold a complex portrait of multiple risk factors related to heart disease and stroke including cigarette smoking, elevated cholesterol and poor diet, hypertension and excessive salt intake, family history, diabetes, inactivity and obesity.

Stroke was shown to be especially sensitive to hypertension and tobacco use.

The major cancers each have their own patterns of risk and slowly each of those was worked out.

Before we proceed to talk about each of these illnesses and their effect on the public's health it is important to look at the forces that helped to identify and promote efforts to deal with these problems. The three most important of these are the American Lung Association (ALA), the American Heart Association (AHA) and the American Cancer Society (ACS).

The American Lung Association began life in 1904 as the National Association for the Study and Prevention of Tuberculosis. The Arkansas Chapter played a vital role by providing money through the Christmas Seal programs, lobbying efforts that had a major impact on the development of the Sanatorium in Boonville and support of other TB programs in the state. Their national research efforts in the 1930s and 1940s into the use of X-ray and TB skin tests helped to identify TB at a much earlier stage. In the 1940s and 1950s, they provided a number of fellowships and large research grants that increased the number of well-trained lung doctors in the United States; these men and women then led many of the fights against smoking

and other occupational air hazards. The ALA's leadership in the tobacco war is well documented and it did not stop with the Surgeon General Report in 1964. Since that time they have led the way in advancing clean air legislation, smoking cessation and reducing the impact of tobacco on our society.

The American Heart Association began in 1915. Heart disease in that day was like cancer – essentially a death sentence; any treatment revolved around bed rest and waiting for the inevitable. In the pre-penicillin days rheumatic heart disease caused by untreated streptococcal infections was common. As life expectancy began to increase, more and more people began suffering from coronary artery disease. By the 1940s, coronary artery disease was the major cause of death and the American Heart Association took on a far more public face. With a federal grant and funds from the AHA, the Arkansas Board of Health, the American Heart Association, and the University of Arkansas Medical Center established a heart evaluation clinic at the Medical Center in the late 1940s. Like the Lung Association the most important activities of the Heart Association have revolved around research, public and professional education and fund raising.

The American Cancer Society had its beginnings in 1912. Growth was slow at first but by the middle of the 1920s, there were 700 chapters across the country. The early focus was on education; "What Everyone Should Know About Cancer" was one of their early and well received pamphlets. The men and women of this organization were masters at fundraising; in 1926 the John D. Rockefeller Foundation donated $125,000 to one of their campaigns. In 1937 when President Roosevelt signed the National Cancer Institute Act, four of the Society's directors were on the six person Advisory Board for the Institute. This act provided funds for each of the states to develop Cancer Commissions. As in earlier days the American Federation of Women's Clubs was intimately involved in the activities of the Cancer Society. In 1936 they formed a Woman's Field Army complete with uniforms to raise money for cancer research especially related to cancer of the breast and uterus. By 1937 the Arkansas Federation took up the cause led by Mrs. F.L. Lake of Hot Springs. This group promoted free screening clinics, fund raising and educational programs. In 1957 the Arkansas Field Army changed its name to the American Cancer Society Arkansas Branch. By the 1950s, the ACS engaged in a campaign encouraging women to have Pap smears and in the 1970s they turned their attention to breast cancer and mammography.

Common to all three of these organizations is a strong emphasis on research—looking for causes and solutions, public and professional education and fund raising to make a strong case for change. Few would argue that all three groups have helped to develop a broad-based constituency for the public's health.

In Arkansas, screening for cancer began as the result of the formation of the Arkansas Cancer Commission in 1945. In one of the truly successful cooperative efforts between the Board of Health and the Arkansas Medical Society, a series of Cancer Clinics were set up around the state. Over the first five years 4,471 cases were treated, 933 were cervical. By 1955 breast, lung, colon and prostate were the most common reported cancers other than skin cancer. The Bowie-Miller Cancer Clinic in Texarkana was the first to get involved in the use of

Pap Smears. By 1957 they reported the results of the first 10 years of their operation and indicated they were using Pap smears on a routine basis; this was not true in the other cancer clinics around the state. Pap smears had been developed by Dr. George Papanicolaou. In 1943 he published a book called "Diagnosis of Uterine Cancer by the Vaginal Smear" and within two decades it was the most widely used screening method in the world. After the 1957 report by the Bowie-Miller Clinic in Texarkana, the other clinics began to increase their usage. By 1962, the University of Arkansas Medical Center was requested to develop a school of cytotechnology to train technical personal primarily to read Pap smears. In the 1960s, only about 30 percent of American women got a Pap smear but by the 1980s that number was greater than 80 percent. In 1962 the American Cancer Society began a national campaign promoting yearly evaluation and Pap smears. In 1975 through a special grant from the National Institute of Health, the Arkansas Health Department provided 35,000 exams and Pap smears in one year for low income women. In the last 40 years, the mortality rate of cervical cancer has dropped by 71 percent and would be much lower if all women got their Pap smears.

The next cancer that fell under the gun was breast cancer. Mammography has a long and complex history dating back to the first uses of the x-ray. Researchers in the late 1950s confirmed that the procedure had merit but it wasn't until 1960 that Dr. Robert Egan at M.D. Anderson in Houston developed a special x-ray film, carefully studied several hundred patients from x-ray to surgery and confirmed an astonishing degree of accuracy. In 1962 the Cancer Control Division of the U.S. Public Health Department with the American College of Radiology sponsored a reproducibility study where they confirmed his work. In addition, they indicated that a radiologist and their technicians could be taught the technique in a five day course. As early as 1969, Dr. Wilma Diner, a radiologist at the University of Arkansas Medical School, presented a paper to the Arkansas Medical Society encouraging the use of mammography. By 1976 the American Cancer Society officially recommended the procedure and began promoting it.

Prior to 1969 and the invention of the fiber-optic flexible colonoscope, the diagnosis of cancer of the colon was quite difficult; almost always the first sign of cancer was bleeding. It was already known that most cancer of the colon arose from otherwise benign polyps. The new scopes allowed for visual inspection of the colon and removal of polyps if present. Prior to the new scope the only means available were rigid scopes that only visualized a small portion of the colon and barium enemas which were notoriously inaccurate. Unlike the Pap smear or the mammogram the scope required a good deal of additional training and because of this it would lag behind the other screening procedures.

Cancer of the prostate like the colon is somewhat difficult to evaluate and the screening procedures including digital rectal exam and the PSA test are imprecise. Prior to 1980 the digital rectal exam was the only test available. When the PSA became available it was thought to be an excellent test for the evaluation of prostate cancer. The problem is that the PSA (prostate specific antigen) is simply a marker for growing prostate tissue and cannot differentiate between normal and abnormal tissue. It is still used as part of the evaluation but is slowly falling into disfavor.

Lung cancer kills more people than all of the other cancers listed above. With the reduction in smoking the numbers for both men and women dying of the disease are beginning to fall. The difficulty is that a good screening test for cancer of the lung is not yet available and because of this most lung cancer is not found until it has spread. If discovered in a localized state, the five-year survival rate is 80 percent; since there is no generally available mass screening that will pick the disease up earlier, the five year survival rate is approximately 17 percent.

And now for the report card, where does Arkansas stand?

Nationally cancer of cervix has a 90 percent five-year survival rate but in Arkansas the number is at about 71.2 percent. The primary reason is lack of Pap smears among black females; 50 percent of cases of cancer of cervix are found after the cancer has spread.

According to the American Cancer Society, breast cancer has an 89 percent five-year survival and in Arkansas the number is 88.7 percent.

The national five-year survival rate for colon cancer is approximately 62 percent and in Arkansas the number is at 64 percent. As with cervical cancer the reason for both of these numbers being low is because 50 percent of the time when the disease is first diagnosed it has spread regionally or distantly from where it started.

Prostate cancer nationally has a 99 percent survival rate for five years despite not having a good screening test; Arkansas is at 98.8 percent.

Lung cancer has an overall five-year survival rate of 17 percent and in Arkansas the number 15.2 percent.

Breast and prostate cancer have a high five-year survival rate. The only way to survive lung cancer is don't get it in the first place and the best way is to use primary prevention—don't smoke. For both cancer of the colon and cancer of the cervix, there are effective preventive health strategies and significant parts of the population are not pursuing them.

In dealing with heart disease and stroke, it is important to note that according to the National Institutes of Health, the death rate from heart disease has dropped by 76 percent since 1963 and the death rate from stroke has dropped by 78 percent. A large part of that drop can be laid at the feet of an effective smoking cessation campaign on the part of state and national organizations begun in 1965. As of 2011, only 21.2 percent of adult Americans smoked, however, close to 27 percent of Arkansans continue to smoke; this in spite of an aggressively pursued Clean Air Act limiting where they can smoke indoors and a very high cost of cigarettes. It is clear that effective blood pressure control has a dramatic and almost immediate impact on the risk of stroke. A number of new families of drugs for the treatment of hypertension have come on the market since the early 1970s and this has had an impact; sadly, Arkansas has the highest stroke mortality in the United State. It is clear from the Framingham Study and the Seven Country study that elevated LDL Cholesterol (bad cholesterol) is a significant risk factor for heart disease as are diabetes, inactivity and obesity; lowering the LDL with exercise, diet and cholesterol-lowering drugs effectively reduces the risk. Obesity has skyrocketed in Arkansas with 66 percent of the state being overweight or obese and as obesity has risen so has diabetes.

CHAPTER NINE
A NEW CENTURY WITH NEW PROBLEMS

The 20th century saw dramatic changes in the patterns of health and disease in Arkansas. Yellow fever, tuberculosis, malaria, smallpox, hookworm, pellagra, polio, typhoid, and various common childhood diseases such as measles, mumps and diphtheria had all responded to effective public health strategies. High infant and maternal mortality dropped substantially in the second half of the 20th century; at the turn of the 21st century, Arkansas's numbers were still higher than the national average but national and state numbers were continuing to improve. Clean water, safe milk and food and good sewer systems improved the lives of most of the citizens of Arkansas. Vigilant efforts in dealing with air, water and soil pollution, though not perfect, were having an impact.

The lines between the public and private health communities have been blurred. With the emergence of potentially effective strategies for dealing with heart disease, stroke, cancer and diabetes, parts of public health have shifted their focus to individual intervention. At the same time the private health care community has begun a shift toward risk factor modification and disease prevention.

The practice of private medicine and its impact on the public's health has changed substantially since the 1960s.

One area of significant change was the proliferation of medicines to treat various ailments— the treatment of hypertension, diabetes, heart disease and common infectious diseases lead the list. At the end of the 1960s, there were only five drugs for hypertension: a couple of diuretics (water pills), guanethidine, methyldopa and reserpine. With the exception of the diuretics these drugs are no longer used primarily because each of them had dreadful side effects. In the 1970s and 1980s, four new families of drugs were introduced with several drugs in each family. Insulin was introduced in the 1920s for the treatment of diabetes and in the early 1960s tolbutamide (Orinase) was introduced as an oral agent for the treatment of diabetes. As with the anti-hypertensive drugs, the 1970s and 1980s saw several new families of medicine for the treatment of diabetes. In the 1960s heart disease was still at a very primitive state. There was no such thing as a coronary care unit; if one was having a heart attack the treatment was to relieve the pain and put the patient to bed. Congestive heart failure was a common problem brought on by repeated heart attacks, uncontrolled hypertension and valvular disease of the heart. The treatment was rest, diuretics and digitalis. Interestingly digitalis, a derivative of the purple foxglove, was one of the herbal holdovers that had been around for 200 years. The use of antibiotics had skyrocketed after World War II and resistant bacteria quickly began to emerge. As with the other drug categories, the 1970s and 1980s saw a proliferation of antibiotic therapies aimed at these resistant bugs.

The surgeon's art had steadily improved for most of the 20th century. Each war saw improvements in technique and anesthesia. The last few decades of the 20th century saw the emergence of increasing subspecialties and the advent of minimally invasive surgical techniques and procedures.

Prior to the 1960s, "getting a physical" was not part of the norm of everyday medicine. Physicals had their beginning in the early 20th century. These physicals were of two varieties: the first was essentially a fitness for duty exam used by the shipping and rail companies and the second type were executive physicals done at the behest of Metropolitan Life Insurance Company when they were asked to insure the life of a high-dollar company boss. In the 1960s, what an individual got as a physical depended a great deal on whom he asked. In Little Rock, Dr. Alfred Kahn, editor of the *Arkansas Medical Society Journal*, would put the patient in the hospital, do three days of tests including every test he could think of and repeat the exam once a year. If the physician was Dr. Frank McGuire of Augusta, he looked in the ears, nose and throat, listened to the chest and, if he was not in a hurry, felt the abdomen. In each case, the physician signed off as having done a physical; in neither case were the exam results credible. The second half of the 20th century saw the development of risk factor profiles, Pap smears, mammography and colonoscopy. In the last 20 years there has been a slow evolution toward a more rational approach based on age, sex and risk profile focused on preventing disease.

The end of the 20th century and the beginning of the 21st century saw the emergence of a number of new unanticipated issues that demanded public health's attention.

A NEW THREAT—HIV

The first of these was the emergence of HIV/AIDS.

HIV/AIDS (Human Immunodeficiency Virus/Acquired Immunodeficiency Syndrome) is two different problems created by a lentivirus. HIV simply implies infection with the virus and AIDS is the condition caused by the virus. Once infected the individual often progresses to failure of the immune system allowing opportunistic infections and cancer and death. When first recognized

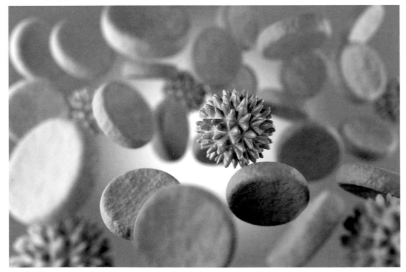

AIDS WAS FIRST RECOGNIZED IN THE UNITED STATES IN NEW YORK AND CALIFORNIA IN 1981. THE FIRST CASE IN ARKANSAS WAS A YOUNG MAN WHO DIED OF AN AIDS-RELATED PNEUMONIA IN 1983.

it was almost always fatal. AIDS was first recognized in the United States in New York and California in 1981.The first case in Arkansas was a young man who died of an AIDS-related pneumonia in 1983. By 1988 there were 126 cases in the state. Among the early cases almost all were men who had sex with men.

Ryan White was a young boy with hemophilia from Indiana who acquired HIV from a blood transfusion and developed AIDS in the late 1980s. He became the poster boy for dealing with AIDS; in August 1990, four months after his death, Congress passed The Ryan White Comprehensive AIDS Resources Emergency (CARE) Act. The act is the United States' largest federally funded program for people living with HIV/AIDS. It provides funds to improve the quality of life and availability of services for low-income victims with AIDS.

In 1996, researchers at an International AIDS Conference in Vancouver demonstrated that three-drug antiviral therapy showed rapid improvement in patients. It was quickly incorporated into clinical practice and rapidly showed impressive benefit with a 60 to 80 percent decline in rates of AIDS and death.

In that same year Arkansas began participating in the federally funded AIDS drug assistance program. In 2000, despite his own publicly stated reactions to the gay and lesbian community, Governor Huckabee signed a bill allowing state dollars to be used for HIV medication for low-income individuals.

Through September 2011, there have been 8,086 cases of AIDS in Arkansas with approximately 2,000 deaths. There are at this point about 5,500 people living with HIV/AIDS in the state with 300 new cases a year, 75 percent are in men who have sex with men, and the majority of the new cases are in African-American males. The most significant problem for the public's health is that 60 percent of those who are infected are not presently under treatment.

TOO MUCH OF A GOOD THING—OBESITY

Another of the problems that manifest itself in the last decades of the 20th century was the problem of obesity. Problems of nutrition and malnutrition are not new to the state of Arkansas. As late as the Depression and the Drought of 1930, pellagra and protein/calorie malnutrition were recurring problems among the rural poor. As early as the 1960s, it became apparent that we as a people were getting bigger and obesity was becoming a major health problem.

Accurately measuring for obesity has always been problematic. Prior to the 1980s, the Metropolitan Life Insurance height and weight tables were used as the gold standard. The Body Mass Index (BMI), a tool used to estimate body fat based on height and weight, replaced those tables in the 1980s. A calculated BMI of 18.5 or less is considered underweight, 18.5 to 25 is considered normal, 25-30 is considered overweight and greater than 30 is considered obese.

There were few accurate records for height and weight kept during the 19th century except for military academy cadets. Using these records researchers have calculated that these young men had amazingly low BMI's with an

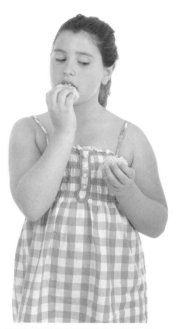

"CHILDREN HAVE NEVER BEEN GOOD AT LISTENING TO THEIR ELDERS BUT THEY HAVE NEVER FAILED TO IMITATE THEM."
JAMES BALDWIN.

average of 20.5. The numbers did not vary greatly during the 19th century but began to show a rise after World War I. By World War II the average had risen to 22.5 and by 1980 to 24.

In 1959, the first National Health Examination Survey evaluating obesity in the United States was performed. At that time 45 percent of American adults were overweight or obese. By 2008 two-thirds of Americans were overweight or obese; Arkansas's numbers are comparable.

At the same time the numbers were rising in adults, the numbers in children have followed suit. In 1960, approximately four percent of children were obese and that number has now grown to greater than 15 percent with another 16 percent of children in the overweight range. In addition, when children are overweight or obese, there is a three out of four chance they will be obese as an adult.

What is the reason for this epidemic of obesity? There are a number of factors that have played a role but relative affluence and inactivity are probably the most important. The emergence of the internal combustion engine, electricity and labor saving devices has resulted in a reduction of physical work and more inactivity. Paradoxically, poverty may play a significant role. A working mother with little money and time may choose a high calorie fast food at lower cost. The last half of the 20th century saw the increasing availability of supersized fast-food and rapidly prepared foods.

If the problem of obesity were simply one of aesthetics, it might be easy to overlook however that is not the case. Overweight adults and children pay a major penalty in long-term illness. Type II diabetes is becoming increasingly common in adults and children. Cardiovascular disease and hypertension are aggravated by and compounded by obesity. Orthopedic problems are dramatically increased in both adults and children. There are estimates that this generation of children may have a lifespan shortened by 10 years as opposed to their parents.

In the 1990s the U.S. Surgeon General and the various state public health organizations across the U.S. began to look for strategies to deal with this and other chronic diseases processes that are aggravated by personal choices and negative cultural norms.

In 2003, Arkansas Act 1220 became the first law in the nation to attempt to combat the epidemic of childhood obesity using a widespread community approach including families, schools, churches and the greater community. The law combating childhood obesity was created with the cooperation of a number of key legislators especially Speaker of the House Hershel Cleveland, the Arkansas Health Department and the Arkansas Department of Education.

In 2007, the Arkansas Coalition for Obesity Prevention was formed following in the footsteps of organizations like the Arkansas Federation of Women's Clubs, Heart Association, the Cancer Society, and the Lung Association. Part of their goal is to create a positive cultural norm both for parents and their children. Identifying the problem and educating the public have been among the most important tasks. Changing the cultural norm is slowly having an impact. Governor Mike Huckabee in the early 2000s developed personal health problems. In response, he lost 100 pounds and became a devotee of healthy practices encouraging a healthier lifestyle. Identifying children in schools with high BMIs has forced many parents to face the truth that both they and their children were at risk. Reducing high sugar content foods and serving size in schools has been mandated in public schools. Encouraging more regular physical activity in the school day clearly is an important part of this equation.

Will these efforts work? The answer is that no one knows for sure however in the last several years there are some encouraging statistics suggesting the problem of childhood obesity may be leveling off and in some areas decreasing.

TRAUMA SYSTEM

In 2013, injury is the leading cause of death among everyone age one to 44—motor vehicle accidents, firearms and suffocation lead the list. In the over 65 age group, falls are near the top of the list.

These numbers are nothing new. As early as 1958, the Arkansas Bureau of Vital Statistics reported the same issues. What became apparent in the 1990s was that Arkansas had a 30 percent higher overall fatality rate per injury than the nation as a whole and the state had an 82 percent higher fatality rate for motor vehicle accidents. In 2008, Arkansas was cited as having the worst system of emergency care in the U.S. Prior to 2009, Arkansas was the only state in the union without a designated trauma center and one of only three states without a trauma system.

The first time this rose to the level of major concern was in 1975 when the legislature created the first EMS (Emergency Medical Services) regulation. From 1975 to 2007, several attempts were made to create an organized system of emergency care; most floundered because of lack of funding. In 2008, Governor Mike Beebe provided $200,000 to create an "emergency dashboard." This facility is an electronic communication facility that expedites the transfer of the injured from one hospital to another. In 2009, the legislature passed the Trauma System Act and appropriated $25 million a year as a result of increasing the excise tax on tobacco to establish and fund the operation. The acute trauma system revolves around a series of four levels of hospitals with level one being the least sophisticated and level four the most. Trauma personnel talk about the "golden hour"—the golden hour is the amount of time from moment of injury until the person is in the hands of someone who can provide definitive care. By December 2012, there were 58 facilities that had signed on to the system with a number of other facilities having submitted applications. A statewide communication systems and upgrading EMS pre-hospital care have been two other elements to this system. As with any effort related to the public's health education, prevention and rehabilitation are integral parts of this network

If other states are any reflection, it may be as long as seven to 10 years before statistical data demonstrates the effectiveness of this system.

A DANGEROUS ENEMY—METH

Alcohol and other street drugs have had a presence in Arkansas since the arrival of man. Prior to the 20th century, there was essentially no control on the manufacture, distribution or use of any of these products. The Clean Food and Drug Act of 1906 was the first federal statute that dealt with narcotic containing products and required the labeling of dangerous ingredients. The Harrison Act of 1914 made the use of opiates illegal except by prescription from a physician. The prohibition of alcohol came and went in the second to fourth decade of the 20th century. In the mid-1950s, President Eisenhower signaled that a war on drugs was coming and in 1970 President Nixon declared the war. Drug usage has waxed and waned for the last century—in the 1950s, heroin and opiates were the drugs of choice; in the 1960s, it was cannabis and hallucinogens, with the 1970s came cocaine, the 1980s saw crack cocaine and the 1990s belonged to methamphetamines.

Arkansas began to see the emergence of an epidemic of methamphetamines in the mid-1990s. The drug itself has been around for a long time; it was first manufactured as early as 1879. In the 1960s, the pharmaceutical industry and the medical profession embraced this class of drugs in a number of forms; amphetamines-like drugs were used for attention span deficient disorder, as nasal decongestants, in the treatment of narcolepsy and as weight control products. It became apparent by the late 1960s that products like Benzedrine (Bennies) had a great deal of abuse potential.

One of the problems with methamphetamine (meth) is that it can be produced using a simple formula and common ingredients in the kitchen. The most important ingredient is the drug pseudoephedrine, a common over-the-counter decongestant. In 1993, the Arkansas Crime Lab reported destroying 16 clandestine meth labs. In 2004, they destroyed more than 2,000 of these labs.

Meth is a stimulant that produces a high that can last for many hours; it is highly addictive and tends to be associated with increased risk of depression, suicide, paranoia, weight loss and malnutrition.

In the early 2000s, 30 percent of the meth produced and used in Arkansas was created in home meth labs. The other 70 percent came from super labs in California and northern Mexico. As the epidemic progressed, the Arkansas court system became inundated with drug crimes; it was apparent that the war on drugs was not working.

In 2005 it was estimated that 74,000 persons in the state suffered from some form of drug addiction or abuse; 151,000 had a problem with alcohol abuse or addiction.

In 2005, the Federal Combating Methamphetamine Act was passed placing restrictions on the availability of pseudoephedrine in drug and groceries stores. This created an immediate drop in the number of illegal home labs discovered and destroyed for the years 2005 to 2008. In 2011 Arkansas passed its own version of the pseudoephedrine restriction laws; similar but more restrictive laws were passed in Oregon and Mississippi and the results have been promising.

Nationally and statewide, drug courts that focused on therapeutic intervention as opposed to jail time have shown a degree of effectiveness.

Arkansas is among the top 10 states in the country with teenagers using prescription pain relievers for non-medical use. For the last three years, the Drug Enforcement Agency, local law enforcement and the Arkansas Department of Health have sponsored Drug Take Back Programs. In September 2012, 5,263 locations across the nation reported collecting 244 tons of old prescription drugs for destruction. On one Saturday afternoon in the fall of 2011, the town of Sherwood, Arkansas collected 66,000 pills and among them 1,400 hydrocodone and 1,000 oxycontin tablets. In 2011, Governor Beebe signed into law the Arkansas's Electronic Prescription Monitoring Program (PMP) as an attempt to enhance prescription monitoring to ensure legitimate use of controlled substances in health care and curtail abuse. This program is being carried out by the Arkansas Department of Health.

FIGHTING TOOTH DECAY

In the 1950s, fluoridation of water had shown dramatic results in the reduction of dental cavities in those communities who availed themselves of the technology. Despite reassurance from the scientific community and the strong backing of the Arkansas Health Department, the Arkansas Dental Association and the Arkansas Medical Society, there was a significant negative reaction to fluoridation in Arkansas during the second half of the 20th century. In February 2010, the Pew Center for the States, the DentaQuest Foundation and the Kellogg Foundation released a study of state efforts to provide low-income children with basic dental care; Arkansas got an F. Dental caries are the most common preventable problem of children in Arkansas. Fluoridation, dental sealants and good dental hygiene would make it possible

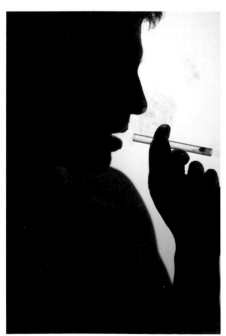

IN 1993, THE ARKANSAS CRIME LAB RE-PORTED DESTROYING 16 CLANDESTINE METH LABS. IN 2004, THEY DESTROYED MORE THAN 2,000 OF THESE LABS.

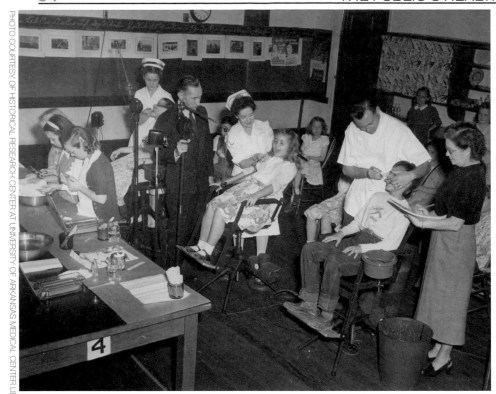

DESPITE REASSURANCE FROM THE SCIENTIFIC COMMUNITY AND THE STRONG BACKING OF THE ARKANSAS MEDICAL SOCIETY, THERE WAS A SIGNIFICANT NEGATIVE REACTION TO FLUORIDATION IN ARKANSAS DURING THE SECOND HALF OF THE 20TH CENTURY.

for most Arkansas children to reach adulthood with no cavities. In 2011, the Arkansas Legislature passed Act 359 that mandated fluoridation of all water systems serving greater than 5,000 people; the goal was to reach 87 percent of the population.

PREPARING FOR THE WORST

As a response to the Cold War in the 1950s and 1960s a system of civil defense was created across the U.S. to deal with the threat of military attack and natural disasters. The beginnings of this system dated back to the two World Wars and Korea but with the advent of intercontinental ballistic missiles armed with nuclear warheads civil defense took on a whole new meaning. Now, places like Arkansas were no longer isolated from the rest of the world in any sense at all. A missile launched in the middle of the Soviet Union could strike Little Rock, Fort Smith or Augusta in 30 minutes. In the 1950s, communities and families in the country lived with this specter and began to build bomb shelters that could be used for the threat of a nuclear disaster or naturally occurring storms. In 1953, the State Civil Defense Agency was created and located in the Arkansas State Capitol in Little Rock. The Agency was soon moved from the Capitol to Camp Robinson in 1955 and in 1957 to Conway because of its distance from Little Rock in the event of a nuclear strike.

For a rural state that is not densely populated, Arkansas has always had a high fatality rate per storm and there are a number of explanations for that. One is the general lack of basements in homes and less-than-sturdy homes in many areas. Unlike the states in Tornado Alley to our west much of Arkansas has mountainous terrain and often it is hard to identify a storm bearing a tornado until it is on top of you. One of the most important elements of effective disaster response is early warning. Prior to World War II the most common mechanism of early warning was church bells. During World War II the electric powered siren came into wide use and by the 1970s were commonplace even in small towns in Arkansas.

In 1961, President Kennedy created the Office of Civil Defense and charged it with developing more sophisticated shelter programs, chemical, biological and radiological warfare defense programs and an enhanced system of early warning that extended down to the individual family.

Part of the thinking process during the Cold War was that major population centers would be struck with nuclear weapons destroying health care infrastructure and because of this in the mid-1960s Civil Defense Emergency Hospitals were developed and placed around the United States. There were 3,000 of these units deployed around the country and 17 scattered across Arkansas. Each of these hospital units weighed 24,000 pounds and was contained in 360 crates for easy transportation. Each unit had its own lab, x-ray, pharmacy, surgical suite, a portable power unit and enough expendable supplies to last for 30 days.

It was the responsibility of the State Board of Health to administer and train for the use of these facilities. In 1965 a second phase to this program was instituted to teach non-medical people a form of medical-self-help and coordinate this with the use of these facilities.

In the 1970s and 1980s when the threat of atomic war began to diminish, the resources that had been directed at the nuclear threat were re-focused dealing with non-military threats such as breaches at the nuclear power plants and chemical and biological agents housed at the facility at Pine Bluff. For most of the state, the resources such as the early warning siren system were re-directed at dealing with natural disasters such as floods and storms especially tornadoes.

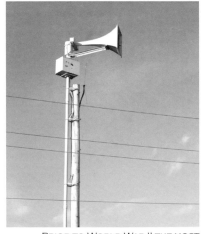

PRIOR TO WORLD WAR II THE MOST COMMON MECHANISM OF EARLY WARNING WAS CHURCH BELLS. DURING WORLD WAR II THE ELECTRIC POWERED SIREN CAME INTO WIDE USE AND BY THE 1970S WERE COMMONPLACE EVEN IN SMALL TOWNS IN ARKANSAS.

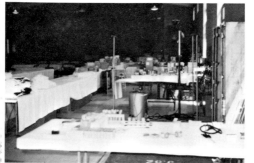

IN THE MID-1960S, 3,000 CIVIL DEFENSE HOSPITALS WERE DEPLOYED AROUND THE COUNTRY AND 17 SCATTERED ACROSS ARKANSAS. EACH OF THESE HOSPITAL UNITS WEIGHED 24,000 POUNDS AND WAS CONTAINED IN 360 CRATES FOR EASY TRANSPORTATION. EACH UNIT HAD ITS OWN LAB, X-RAY, PHARMACY, SURGICAL SUITE, A PORTABLE POWER UNIT AND ENOUGH EXPENDABLE SUPPLIES TO LAST FOR 30 DAYS.

From the 1970s to 2001, emergency management and preparedness services in Arkansas went through a series of changes including several name changes and increasing responsibility. It was ultimately named the Arkansas Department of Emergency Management and all of the disaster planning was subsumed by one organization. The Emergency Medical support function of ADEM is provided by the Arkansas Health Department.

On September 11, 2001 a new and major threat was added to the role of the emergency medical support, bioterrorism: agents such as Anthrax, Smallpox, Ebola, weapons-grade tularemia, ricin and poison gases.

In 2002, Dr. Joe Bates enticed Dr. Bill Mason, a homegrown expert in lung and infectious disease, to manage the emergency response branch of the State Health Department. Bill was raised in the tiny town of Norphlet, Arkansas in the middle of the oil fields and refineries. He clearly remembers the air, water and soil pollution that dominated that area in the pre-EPA days and because of this has always had a strong interest in public health. As a young lung specialist in central Arkansas, he had worked for Doctors Bates and Stead in the TB Chest Clinics for a number of years.

When Dr. Paul Halverson became head of the Department of Health in 2005, he brought with him a great deal of expertise and interest in emergency management. With his encouragement, Dr. Mason and his branch developed a state of the art Emergency Operations Center (EOC) in the basement of the main Health Department building on West Markham in Little Rock. When the building was completed and occupied in 1968 the space that now contains the EOC was the bomb shelter for essential state officials.

In the last several years, the EOC has been activated for a number of disaster events. The most important of these was for Hurricane Katrina and the massive number of refugees. Seventy-thousand refugees were brought into the state, processed into camps where they were allowed to stabilize, their health care and creature comforts were dealt with and eventually they were out-processed. The project extended over a period of several months but most of the heavy work was in the first eight weeks. It was a project that required the full cooperation of everyone from the governor down to the volunteers who worked in the camps. It was the first such major event of disaster relief since the Flood of 1937.

On March 29, 2013 a 65-year-old Exxon pipeline carrying Canadian crude oil ruptured, spilling thousands of gallons of oil into a residential area in Mayflower, Arkansas. Within a short period of time, the flow of oil was stopped, the residents were evacuated and the spilled oil was contained. The EPA, ADEM and other state agencies responded quickly. It became the role of the Health Department personnel to begin evaluating any impact on the air and water and make recommendations. There has been conflicting information as to any residual effect on air and water, but the long term health consequences are yet to be determined.

Except for those citizens who live in the immediate area of the spill the significance of this spill is what it highlights. Many metropolitan areas like Little Rock depend on surface water impoundments like Lake Maumelle and Lake Winona. There is a large old pipeline in the catchment area of Lake Maumelle and if it ruptured could quickly foul the water supply for central Arkansas.

From the health standpoint the biggest worry that Dr. Mason and his cohorts have is a major earthquake along the New Madrid fault and the disruptions it could cause in the power and transportation grids; the impact of transport up and down the Mississippi and the potential for massive oil spills in Arkansas, Tennessee, Mississippi and Louisiana.

THE SAD FACTS OF RURAL HEALTH

It seems fitting that we should end on the subject of rural health.

Since the creation of the Arkansas Territory in 1819, there have been significant health disparities between rich and poor, white and black, city and the country. In 2013, Arkansas continues to deal with these legacies of the past plus a number of new problems.

In 1900, 90 percent of Arkansas's population lived in rural areas, by 1940 that had dropped to 80 percent. The 1950s and 1960s saw a significant out-migration of population from the entire state, but a disproportionate amount of this loss was from the rural areas. In the last part of the 20th century the population of the state began rebounding, but the rural areas and especially the Delta continued to drop. In 2009, just over 46 percent of Arkansans lived in a rural setting.

One of the difficulties with discussing rural health in Arkansas is that there are several different types of rural areas in the state. These divisions fall roughly along the various geographic regions. The Mississippi Delta in eastern Arkansas is by far the poorest and least healthy, the Gulf Coastal Plain of south Arkansas is slightly better but not by much. The Mountain Highlands including the Ozarks and Ouachitas are next up the ladder on the health scale. These rural areas stand in sharp contrast to the urban areas of Central Arkansas, Northwest Arkansas, a small segment of Northeast Arkansas and Miller county in the southwest corner of the state.

Looking back to the beginning of the 20th century when public health and the private health care community began to take on some legitimacy most of the emphasis was focused on population centers. The idyllic myth of clean disease-free living in the country in contrast to dirty cities had its origins back at the beginnings of the industrial age when clean water and sewer systems were not part of the social contract. The negative penalty for living in large communities began to disappear by the middle of the 19th

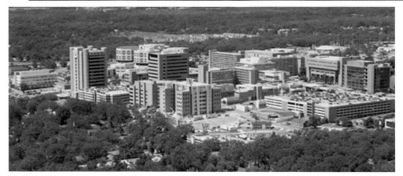

IN 1974 THE AREA HEALTH EDUCATION CENTER PROGRAM AT UAMS WAS CREATED WITH CENTERS IN FORT SMITH, PINE BLUFF AND EL DORADO. BY 1980, THERE WERE THREE ADDITIONAL CENTERS IN FAYETTEVILLE, JONESBORO AND TEXARKANA.

century. Except in times of crisis like floods, droughts and storms people in the country were left to their own devices. That changed in the 1930s as the Arkansas Board of Health developed an increasing presence in many of the small rural communities around the state. At the same time the number of tools at the disposal of rural physicians began to expand their usefulness beyond hand holding, delivering babies and emergency surgery.

The collection of accurate vital statistics beginning in the 1940s began to highlight the health problems faced by Arkansans as well as the disparities. Especially important in those early days were communicable diseases such as syphilis, various childhood diseases and maternal and child care. The New Deal legislation of the 1930s created a number of programs related to venereal diseases and maternal and child care that injected large amounts of money into rural health.

With the out-migration of the 1950s and 1960s, health care access increasingly became a problem in rural areas. Health care access for the African-American population had always been limited, but now the access problem crossed the racial boundaries. The rural physician and nursing populations were aging and no one was replacing them. At the University Medical Center in Little Rock there was a strong emphasis on training specialists who tended to settle in larger communities. Dr. Ben Saltzman, head of the Arkansas Health Department in the 1970s, was a rural physician from Mountain Home, Arkansas; as early as the 1950s, he began publishing articles on the plight of rural health in Arkansas.

In the early 1950s the Arkansas Legislature passed the Peebles Act that required the admission committee at the Medical School to use as one of their criteria for acceptance an equitable distribution from each of the legislative districts. That legislature also passed a loan program that could be converted to a scholarship for those physicians who agreed to practice in a community of 2,000 or less.

In 1954 the Winthrop Rockefeller Foundation funded a series of surveys and a pilot project in Perry County, Arkansas. This Rural Medicine Project involved building a clinic, staffing it with a physician and studying the un-met need. The project was a failure and soon collapsed on itself. One of the positive outcomes was a survey that showed that 82 percent of the

population of the state, city and rural, felt there were not enough doctors in their area.

During the 1960s, this became painfully obvious across the United States. The increasing prevalence of private health insurance and the passage of Medicare and Medicaid meant that larger numbers of people were seeking care and there simply weren't enough health care personnel to service everyone. In the late 1960s, the Carnegie Foundation created a commission to study the problem and in 1970 they published their report, Higher Education and the Nation's Health: Policies for Medical and Dental Education. Their studies confirmed what everyone suspected: there weren't enough health care personnel and they weren't in the right places. The commission offered a series of recommendations designed to create a system that put essential health services within one hour of driving time for 95 percent of all Americans.

One of their most far reaching recommendations was the establishment of Area Health Education Centers across the country. These were to be centers of training and health care associated with University Medical Schools in rural areas around the country. A number of studies had shown that the region where a student and resident studies is a strong determinate in where they locate and practice. Based on the commission's findings Congress passed the Comprehensive Health Manpower Training Act that provided funding for the development and operation of these centers.

In the early 1970s, Governor Dale Bumpers authorized the development of a State Health Plan to deal with the health manpower shortage, maldistribution of health care personnel and the problem of access to care especially for those who lived in the rural part of the state. The first of their recommendations was the implementation of an Area Health Education Center system. Other recommendations included the development of an emergency medical services system, the enhancement of UAMS to recruit and train more family physicians and a plan to increase the capabilities of the Arkansas Health Department—expanding nursing services, developing ambulatory care centers in areas of scarcity, expanding dental care, transportation and improving telephone access.

For a second time the admissions committee at UAMS was charged to review the application process—if two applicants for a position had equal credentials, the rural candidate was to be given preference.

In 1971, the medical school launched a three year Family Practice Residency based in Little Rock as an attempt to train and place family practice doctors in rural areas. In 1974, the Area Health Education Center Program was created with centers in Fort Smith, Pine Bluff, and El Dorado; by 1980 there were three additional centers in Fayetteville, Jonesboro, and Texarkana. Each of these locations developed a fully-certified three-year family practice residency, preceptorships for medical students and rotations for internal medicine residents. By 2007 there were two more centers in Mountain Home and Batesville.

The Rural Health Scholarship Program of the early 1950s was not especially successful and in 1974 it was rewritten and expanded; this in conjunction with changes in the medical school admission process and the AHEC programs did result in an increase in the numbers of physicians entering rural areas and being retained.

Every state governor since Winthrop Rockefeller in the late 1960s with the possible exception of Frank White (1981-1983) has pursued solutions to the rural health problem in Arkansas. All of the directors of the Arkansas Health Department have understood the role of ADH in the public's health and especially the rural public's health.

As with Maternal and Infant care, there has been an alphabet-soup of different agencies and programs that have come and gone based on the availability of funding. Two ongoing programs that have had an impact on the public's health are the Center for Rural Health at UAMS and the Office of Rural Health and Primary Care at the ADH. These two programs and the UAMS School of Public Health provide a 21st century framework for the broader problems of rural public health in Arkansas.

The Center for Rural Health at UAMS serves to extend the efforts begun in the 1970s through the AHEC centers at recruitment and retention of health professionals in rural areas, provide telemedicine resources, ongoing education and research into evolving healthcare problems.

The Office of Rural Health and Primary Care, founded in 1991, is an organization that functions as a part of the Center for Local Health at ADH. Its primary function is to coordinate public and private efforts to provide health care to those living in rural areas.

Before we discuss the strategies being pursued in 2013 we need to outline the problems faced on the ground in rural Arkansas.

There are 3 million people who live in the state of Arkansas and almost half live in rural areas. The racial makeup between urban and rural is not dramatically different except for south and east Arkansas where African-Americans make up one-third of the population. There is an increasing percentage of Hispanics in the western counties and estimates are that by 2025 they will be the largest minority in the state. The counties in the Delta and Costal Plains are losing population, school enrollment and jobs at a rapid rate. Arkansas has the second highest poverty rate in the nation at 19 percent and there are pockets in the Delta where the rate is greater than 25 percent.

The average life expectancy in Arkansas is 76 years compared to the national average of 78 years. Benton County in northwest Arkansas has a life expectancy of 79.8 years and there are 17 counties, most in the south and east, with a life expectancy six to 10 years less than Benton County. The areas with the lowest life expectancy have the highest rates of infant mortality, obesity, heart disease, stroke, cancer and diabetes. The African-American population has an overall mortality rate one-third higher than their white counterparts. Access to health care is limited and those who live in rural settings are more likely to be involved in fatal accidents and less likely to have emergency services. Forty-six of the state's counties have only one hospital and 21 counties have no hospital. Medical transportation for emergency or routine care is limited and unpredictable in many areas.

There are a number of components that must be in place to provide care in a rural setting as described above.

The first of these is health care professionals to provide the care. By national standards, every county in the state except for Sebastian County is considered medically underserved. In most parts of rural Arkansas, the numbers of physicians and nurse practitioners is low and decreasing every year. Several different types of organizations have evolved to try and correct this problem.

During the 1960s, the concept of Community Health Centers evolved out of the Johnson War on Poverty. The Office of Economic Opportunity (OEO) originally established "neighborhood health centers" to provide medical services to low-income neighborhoods.

These clinics evolved into federally qualified and funded Community Health Centers. Early on these organizations were funded by grants and have slowly made the evolution to Medicaid and Medicare funding as their primary source of funds. There are 12 federally-qualified Community Health Centers (CHCs) in the state of Arkansas. The stated goal of these centers is to provide equal access to total health care regardless of the ability to pay. The CHCs of Arkansas have a total of 63 full-time equivalent physicians, 27 advanced practitioner nurses, 127 RN/LPNs and 15 full-time equivalent dentists. The largest of these organizations is ARCare (formerly White River Rural Health Cooperative). ARCare is the brainchild of Dr. Steve Collier of Augusta, Arkansas. Raised on the banks of the White River, he attended Baylor for college then returned to UAMS where he got his M.D. degree and followed that up with a three year family practice residency at the AHEC in Pine Bluff. As he was finishing his residency it came to his attention that a group of businessmen and the county judge of his hometown had built a clinic and were looking for a young physician. It didn't take long before he was convinced to give it a try. Early on, the health department in Augusta was struggling and he combined forces with them and their Family Planning efforts. By 1983, the Augusta Clinic extended its range to included Cotton Plant and Des Arc and from that ARCare evolved. As of 2013, ARCare has a presence in 12 different counties in east and east central Arkansas with at least 24 clinics; they have 30 physicians, 18 advanced practitioner nurses and two pharmacists. The decision process to take on a new community is generally a three year process. For the first year, they identified a total of 60 to 90 individuals in the community through a series of meetings seeking their input as to what the medical needs of the community are. The second year is spent planning, raising funds and the third year is devoted to doing something concrete to show that they mean business. Dr. Collier is quick to point out that they do not go into communities and duplicate services; they do not set themselves up as competition for the providers already there.

As he points out each community is different with different perceived needs. In Augusta they built a Wellness Center to help deal with chronic disease, in McCrory they helped to build a new nursing home, in several communities they have enticed an older physician to come to work for them and fold his clinic into their organization. They have an AIDS expert who works with the ADH treating AIDS in rural settings around the state. They have created a collaborative pharmacy project in Kensett with the new pharmacy school in Searcy.

In the years to come, they will have some hard service decisions to make as some of the small communities they serve disappear back into

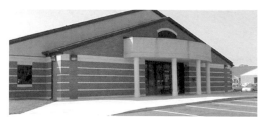

SINCE THE INCEPTION OF THE ARKANSAS BOARD OF HEALTH, LOCAL HEALTH UNITS, LIKE THIS ONE IN SALINE COUNTY, HAVE FORMED THE BACKBONE OF PUBLIC HEALTH.

the countryside.

There are two other types of clinic structures around state that provide similar types of care in underserved areas.

The Rural Health Clinics (RHC) can be public, private, for-profit or not-for-profit. There are 64 of these around the state, usually staffed by an advanced practitioner nurse who is supervised by a physician.

The Arkansas Association of Charitable Clinics was founded in 2004 and pulled together 26 clinics in 22 different counties. These clinics are staffed with volunteer physicians, nurses, pharmacists and clerical staff.

The last 20 years has seen the emergence of telemedicine and the internet allowing remote health personnel such as radiologist, psychiatrists, medical and surgical subspecialists to assist patients and their health care providers in the evaluation and the development of treatment plans for complex problems. They have not been a cure-all but certainly seem to be helping.

Since their inception in the early 20th century local health units have been the bedrock of the public's health. The words of C.E.A. Winslow describing public health as, "the science and art of disease prevention, prolonging life, and promoting health and well-being through organized community effort," have guided the daily work of the public health nurses, doctors, dentists, veterinarians, nutritionists and sanitarians of Arkansas. Often but not always their work has revolved around the medically under-served populations in the state. Their work is seldom glamorous and goes un-recognized until there is a crisis. As of 2008 the Local Health Units of the Arkansas Health Department continue to have a strong presence in rural Arkansas. There were 1,300 personnel employed in providing public health services at the local unit level and 3,500 engaged in providing in-home services.

In 1998, the Health Department created a program called Hometown Health Improvement. The purpose of this program is to assist communities in evaluating and responding to their unique needs. What began as a pilot project in Boone County in 1998 had reached all 75 counties by 2009. Grants and Tobacco Settlement money were used to hire and train 17 BSN trained Registered Nurses to act as Community Health Nurse Specialists in the five different public health regions of the state. In addition to helping communities develop plans of action these nurses work closely with the schools and school health nurses. In the last several years, they have broadened their mission to help deal with childhood obesity and physical inactivity. Health education for both young and old is an important element to improving the overall health in the rural parts of the state.

Since 1987 and the appointment of Dr. Jocelyn Elders as head of the ADH, minority health issues have been front and center in the efforts of public health in Arkansas. As we discussed earlier African-Americans, rural and urban, have a dramatic difference in mortality for most disease states. Of increasing importance is the Hispanic minority many of whom live in rural areas. Increasing emphasis is being placed on language barriers and access to care among these new immigrants. A third minority that acts as a rural population are the Marshallese of northwest Arkansas. In the 1970s, the U.S. allowed a legal migrant population from the Marshall Islands to enter the country as reparation for the nuclear testing in their islands. Approximately 8,000 have settled in the Springdale area. It turned out that they have a high rate of tuberculosis, hepatitis B, syphilis and Hanson's disease (leprosy). Since this migrant population is not eligible for most state and federal aid or assistance, they have provided a rather difficult public health problem.

The next component in the network of rural care is the Critical Access Hospitals. There are a number of problems faced by the population of Arkansas that can't be dealt with in an out-patient setting. For several decades many of the original Hill-Burton hospitals across the U.S. have been forced to close their doors because of increasing financial pressures. With the Medicare Modernization Act of 2003, the designation of Critical Access Hospital was created which provided small rural hospitals cost-based reimbursement and a financial leg up. There are 108 hospitals across the state including 47 acute care hospitals. Twenty-eight of these have been designated as Critical Access Hospitals distributed around the state.

The Arkansas rural transportation system is decentralized and haphazard. Availability of transportation is often quite limited and can present a major barrier to health care. Emergency services are especially critical. Making contact with critical medical personnel that can perform definitive procedures within the "golden hour" after an event or accident is most important. In 2008, there were 120 ambulance companies, 6,000 paramedics and EMTs and 609 ground ambulances in Arkansas. Of the 609 ground ambulances, one-third were greater than seven years old. Seventy percent of those services were privately owned and operating in rural areas. Twenty-three volunteer fire departments provide ambulance service with only minimal training and basic life support. Most EMS air transport was provided by 24 services both private and hospital based. Seventeen of the services were based in-state and seven in our border states of Tennessee, Louisiana, Texas, Oklahoma and Missouri. One of the key components to the new Arkansas Trauma System is to upgrade the ground and air ambulance systems in Arkansas setting new standards, recruiting and training.

Will the Arkansas Department of Health, through its office of Rural Health, local public health services, the Community Health Centers like ARCare, Critical Access Hospitals and an upgraded trauma system with sophisticated EMS services, solve some of the problems of the public's health in rural Arkansas? Based on the past experience over the last 100 years it seems that the probability is high they will. It is also highly probable that before they have time to congratulate themselves another equally dreadful and dramatic problem will present itself.